ABOUT THE AUTHOR

A qualified medical doctor and nutritionist who founded The Food Effect, www.thefoodeffect.co.uk, Dr Michelle Braude runs an innovative nutrition consultancy practice based in North London, as well as a popular online blog in which she shares and explains the health benefits of her favourite recipes.

Born in sunny South Africa and raised in London, Michelle is at the forefront of the future of healthcare. She combines her background in medicine, expertise in the science of nutrition, and passion for cooking and delicious food, to offer a comprehensive and practical service that is unique.

Michelle qualified as a medical doctor (MBBS) from the prestigious University College London (UCL). During her medical studies, she completed a Bachelor of Science (BSc) degree in nutrition at King's College London, as well as carrying out an elective period in gastroenterology at the Whittington Hospital, London. This provided further opportunity for her to increase her knowledge and gain practical experience in the wide range of clinical conditions covered by this area of medicine.

Not long after graduating, Michelle's passion for nutrition prompted her to set up her own nutrition practice, The Food Effect, in 2012. With mounting clinical evidence on the effect of nutrition on health and well-being, Michelle realised she could use her combined knowledge in the fields of medicine and nutrition to help patients with medical conditions, such as high blood pressure, high cholesterol and diabetes, to improve their health through changing their diets. As her unique approach developed, she also began specialising in improving the diets

and optimising the overall health and well-being of people who did not have a medical condition but needed or wanted to lose weight. Within a year, with many happy clients and numerous success stories, the project had become a hugely successful nutrition practice and online business.

Since officially founding The Food Effect, Michelle's reputation and practice have grown rapidly. Her unique expertise in the field of nutrition, teamed with her growing public and online profiles, have resulted in Michelle being a sought-after expert. She is regularly featured as an independent expert in the *Daily Mail*, *Daily Telegraph*, *The Times*, *Hello!*, *Women's Health*, the *Mirror* and *Marie Claire* magazine.

Needless to say, the next logical step was to share her secrets in a book.

Michelle's first book, *The Food Effect Diet* was published in January 2018, and serialised by *The Times* newspaper. It has received amazing feedback and reviews, and first-hand results from many happy readers worldwide.

Michelle has built a highly engaged and ever-growing audience, on her popular Instagram page – @thefoodeffectdr – where she shares all her nutrition tips, advice and delicious recipes on a daily basis.

With a growing interest from many vegan followers online, as well as the success of many vegan clients, Michelle was inspired to write her second book, *The Food Effect Diet Vegan*, which she is so thrilled to share with you here. With both a medical degree and a BSc in nutrition, Michelle is uniquely placed to create an effective, delicious meal plan that is also nutritionally complete and based on proven science – one that will ensure optimal health and long-lasting results.

THE
FOOD
EFFECT
DIET
VEGAN

DR MICHELLE BRAUDE

piatkus

PIATKUS

First published in Great Britain in 2020 by Piatkus

1 3 5 7 9 10 8 6 4 2

A CIP catalogue record for this book
is available from the British Library.

ISBN 978-0-349-42468-2

Typeset in Sabon by M Rules
Printed and bound in Great Britain by Clays Ltd, Elcograf S.p.A.

Papers used by Piatkus are from well-managed forests
and other responsible sources.

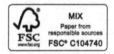

Piatkus
An imprint of
Little, Brown Book Group
Carmelite House
50 Victoria Embankment
London EC4Y 0DZ

An Hachette UK Company
www.hachette.co.uk

www.improvementzone.co.uk

Dedicated to my parents, who raised me to always reach for the stars, and to live every day with gratitude, kindness and positivity. Without you both, nothing in my life would be possible.

CONTENTS

FOREWORD

I feel that I have to open this foreword with a statement, and that statement is: Dr Michelle Braude quite literally changed my life.

After going vegetarian at the age of 12, I transitioned to veganism when I was 26, inspired by the concept of making a real difference to the animals, and after watching many, many videos about the truth of the dairy and egg industries.

As many of us do, I stumbled across an array of vegan YouTubers, small and slim in physique, but who promoted unlimited calories, and promised that if it's vegan, it's good. At this time, I was living in Brussels, Belgium, a country not known for being vegan-friendly and I found myself trying to emulate the examples of my vegan YouTube idols; however, I soon started to put on weight, and became almost obsessed with food. Is it vegan? What shall we have for lunch? Of course I can eat this huge doughnut! How bad can it be, it's vegan?

This pattern carried on for several years. I wasn't happy with my body or my relationship with food. True, going vegan was one of the best decisions I have made, but I felt so disconnected from proper portion sizes and I was always comparing myself to other vegans.

I joined so many Facebook Groups in search of answers, weight-loss tips and help, but the mishmash of advice, as well as the occasional snide remark, made me feel self-conscious and ashamed that I was trying to heal my food issues and lose weight.

As my professional life took off, I found that my eating patterns nose-dived. Working in marketing and PR, time was always of the essence, so most days I was fuelled with coffee, hummus and whatever I could lay my hands on that I could eat at my desk. After running the marketing department for the Veganuary 2019 campaign, I realised that something had to give. I felt that I was running on empty, I was 'tired and wired', always hungry, and dinner time was a combination of half a bottle of wine and a whole load of snacking and pasta. I was, ultimately, lost.

I had connected with Dr Michelle on Instagram through a mutual friend, and after reading her first book, *The Food Effect Diet*, I realised that I needed some proper guidance, so I booked a consultation with her. I haven't looked back since.

Not only have I lost the weight that I was struggling with for years, but my whole relationship with food and my body has shifted. After eating nutritious, balanced meals and snacks, I no longer felt ravenous all the time, and I even had an incredible amount of energy after just Day 2 of the plan. My focus on food turned to become a focus on my life and what I could do to create a business and a lifestyle that served me and would bring balance and wellness into my life again.

Many people think that eating plans are all about losing weight, and yes, if you have some pounds to lose, following a structured regime is most probably going to help you in that regard. But what I loved about *The Food Effect Diet* – and now *The Food Effect Diet Vegan* – is how Dr Michelle navigates the complicated relationships we can have with food (see Chapter 7 about this) and breaks all this information down into digestible chunks.

Do you love wine? Great, you can still drink it. Do you have to eat a piece of chocolate in the evening? You can still do that. The Food Effect lifestyle is exactly that: it fits in with your life, and it makes the results and the mindset shift all the more effective and sustainable.

Dr Michelle brings her scientific and medical knowledge to help people feel their very best, which is why I'm so thrilled to introduce *The Food Effect Diet Vegan*.

With veganism growing at an exponential rate, and often for ethical or environmental reasons, health can end up not being a focus. And this can be perpetuated by dietary advice being sought from those who are not qualified to give it.

Plant-based food is so full of vibrancy and life, and after implementing *The Food Effect Diet Vegan* methodology, I have no doubt that you, too, will feel that you are the best version of yourself while still adhering to your veganism.

Dr Michelle provides a solid education and gentle guidance as she helps you to navigate the supplements you might need, to understand the correct portion of carbohydrates we should be having and to reconnect with the joy of food that makes you thrive, without spending a fortune on fancy schmancy ingredients that you've never heard of – all without depriving yourself.

The recipes in this book are quite simply delectable, and my personal favourites are the Hummus-Stuffed Dates (the perfect afternoon snack) and the Green Bean and Butternut Casserole with Crunchy Peanut Butter Sauce.

After working with Dr Michelle, I've found a whole new lease of life: I'm eating healthy, nutrient-dense food; I've lost weight while still having my favourite treats; and I was inspired to start my own business and realise that I have the power to change my life.

I'll be forever grateful to Dr Michelle, and I'm so excited to see her help many, many more vegans to feel happy, healthy and energised.

Rachida Brocklehurst, vegan entrepreneur, copywriter, PR expert for female entrepreneurs, luxury and vegan-friendly businesses. Previous author at Veganuary and the *Huffington Post*

The Food Effect Diet Vegan

Eat more, weigh less, look and feel better

You don't have to be a vegan to enjoy and benefit from the recipes and guidance contained in this book. The Food Effect Diet Vegan is aimed at:

- Vegans who wish to lose weight or stay slim and improve their overall health, energy levels and vitality.
- Vegans who want science-based dietary advice from a qualified medical doctor and nutritionist.
- Vegans who want simple, easy meal and snack suggestions.
- Vegans who want over 70 new quick-and-easy vegan recipes that are uncomplicated, easy to prepare and waistline-friendly.
- Vegans who want advice on dining out, supplements, exercise and more.
- Non-vegans who wish to lose weight, feel better and give veganism a go.
- Non-vegans who are looking to explore more plant-based ways of cooking and eating without adding extra calories to their diet.
- Non-vegans who wish to cut down on animal-based food for health reasons.

- Anyone who wants to eat in a more environmentally sustainable way.
- Anyone who wants to improve their health and decrease their risk of disease.
- Anyone who wants a wide range of new, delicious and healthy waistline-friendly vegan recipes.
- Anyone who wants to discover new and different foods.
- Anyone who wants to save money (the meals and recipes are super-economical).
- Anyone who wants a structured meal plan and tempting recipes that are simple to prepare, nutritionally balanced and effective for weight loss.

The popularity of veganism is increasing rapidly, and there are more and more vegan recipe books coming out constantly; however, there is very little in the way of weight-loss books that can guide those following a vegan diet to lose weight simply, healthily and effectively, together with providing a guide, a meal plan and recipes to cater to a vegan diet.

In the past year I've received hundreds of messages on social media asking if my original book, *The Food Effect Diet*, which thankfully has shown incredible results, is suitable for vegans. I've also experienced a huge rise in the number of clients I see who are vegan and who want a vegan meal plan for weight loss and improved health and well-being. All this has inspired me to write *The Food Effect Diet Vegan*.

The Food Effect philosophy grew from my desire to teach people how to eat normally and healthily in a way that they can continue for the rest of their lives. It is based on the belief that healthy eating is an essential, pleasurable, colourful and vibrant way of life – and one that can be achieved by everyone, if they are shown how.

In the course of building up a successful nutrition practice, and helping hundreds of happy clients, I developed The Food Effect diet and lifestyle plan to show people how they can eat more, weigh less and both look and feel better, without compromising their lifestyle. Following its success, along with the increasing popularity of veganism, and working with many vegan clients, I wanted to create The Food Effect Diet Vegan – an approach that shows you how to eat more, weigh less, look better and feel better, all while following a vegan lifestyle with ease and enjoyment.

The Food Effect Diet Vegan presents a simple, delicious and satisfying way of eating that sheds weight, boosts energy, lowers cholesterol and blood pressure, and also gives you glowing skin, increased brain power and optimal health and vitality. It teaches the simple secrets of long-term practical success for weight loss for vegans, without requiring you to cut out any more food groups than necessary, such as carbs (yes, even some vegans promote cutting out carbs).

Instead, you'll be encouraged to eat carbs at every meal, have a late-night treat and avoid the faddish routes of cutting out wheat, gluten, carbs or fats. What's more, you'll be allowed to dine out and enjoy coffee, alcohol and dark chocolate from day one, without it compromising your weight-loss goals, or your vegan principles.

What's included?

The Food Effect Diet Vegan comprises:

- Two simple stages – The Food Effect Diet Vegan Attack Phase and The Food Effect Diet Vegan Lifestyle – that are incredibly easy to stick to.
- A wide array of vegan food choices, including surprising sources of good-for-you carbs, proteins and fats.
- Menu options for breakfast, lunch, dinner and snacks based on a variety of taste preferences, lifestyles and nutritional needs.
- Over 70 delicious and easy vegan recipes, plus a complete set

of simple meal ideas for those who don't like to cook or who don't have time to do so.

- Practical, comprehensive food tables, featuring every food group (from vegan proteins, carbs, fruit and vegetables, to beverages, condiments and alcohol), in clear, practical 'Eat this', 'Be careful' and 'Stay away' categories.
- Dietary recommendations – designed with a calorie cap (so that there's no calorie counting involved) to ensure that you achieve your weight-loss goals.
- Plenty of variety to keep things interesting.
- Up-to-the minute tips and advice, including supplement advice and recommendations specifically for vegans to ensure that all your nutritional needs are met.
- Advice on overcoming potential obstacles and individual struggles, including tips on managing cravings and avoiding overeating.

What makes The Food Effect Diet Vegan unique?

These days, we seem to be gluttons for fad diets (I've seen many vegan detoxes, juice cleanses and extreme diets being promoted online), and while they might appear to be a quick-fix solution and lead to weight loss in the short term, over time they slow down your metabolism, are unsustainable and simply cause you to pile the pounds back on straight after you come off them. The Food Effect Diet Vegan approach, in contrast, is based on scientific understanding of human anatomy and physiology, and doesn't change with the tides of fad dieting, juice cleanses, soup diets or vegan detoxes.

In this book I share the simple strategies that I have used to help many vegan clients shed weight and – more importantly – to keep it off, while at the same time improving their health, energy and vitality.

What sets my vegan plan apart from the current swathe of trendy fad diets? There are two major differences:

1. It is nutritionally sound.

2. It is written by a qualified medical doctor and nutritionist who has first-hand results from many vegan clients who have followed this plan.

Easy and nutritious

Simple and effective without being overly complicated, The Food Effect Diet Vegan delivers a painless and proven way to achieve your weight-loss goals and get you on the road to optimal health. It's all about eating more of the right things. That means packing in as much good, wholesome nutrition as possible via delicious healthy vegan meals and snacks, so that there's no room for the bad stuff.

What's more, by eating delicious, wholesome, tasty foods (not celery sticks and lettuce leaves) you won't find the diet difficult to stick to, either, and you certainly won't be expected to go hungry. It's all about making simple changes that don't feel like a sacrifice; for example, swapping crisps for salted popcorn, or switching from unhealthy processed vegan puddings and biscuits to far healthier dark chocolate or my guilt-free vegan desserts. That way you won't ever feel as though you're missing out.

A vegan weight-loss diet is different

Whereas there are countless diet books on the market, most diet books are not vegan or easily adaptable for those following a vegan lifestyle, and there are plenty of vegans who want to lose weight and improve their health.

Most diet and recipe books, including my original *The Food*

Effect Diet book, can be easily adapted to suit a vegetarian diet (for example, by replacing chicken or turkey with eggs or dairy). But for someone who is vegan, it's much more difficult to adapt a non-vegan diet and/or recipe book. Therefore, I have created a diet book specifically for vegans, and also for those who aren't necessarily vegan but who would like to adopt a more plant-based lifestyle (perhaps by eating less meat and fewer animal products) but who need some ideas and inspiration.

Many people assume that being vegan automatically equates with being slim or losing weight, but this is certainly not the case. Although there are endless health (and other) benefits to following a plant-based vegan lifestyle, there are also many challenges. Vegan clients I've seen are often struggling to incorporate enough protein into their diets from real whole-food sources, and, as a result, are eating many highly processed, high calorie, unhealthy vegan products. Additionally, it's easy to go overboard with many, although healthy, vegan-friendly foods – such as nuts, hummus, avocado, olive oil, nut butters, and so on – where the calories can easily add up, making weight gain inevitable. I've seen many vegan clients in such a position, who come to me feeling stuck and confused as to why their 'healthy' vegan diet is making them pile on the pounds. Thankfully, all of them achieved amazing results after their Food Effect consultation, receiving guidance from myself and following their Food Effect Diet Vegan meal plans – all very similar to what is included in this book.

A medically approved approach

I've written *The Food Effect Diet Vegan* based on my first-hand experience as a medical doctor and qualified nutritionist in helping many vegan clients lose weight, as well as incorporating the philosophy of my first book *The Food Effect Diet*, which has received amazing feedback.

The recipes, meal plans and all advice are backed up by

nutritional science and ensure that all your nutritional needs will be met from all the essential food groups. Achieving your weight-loss goals will not come at the expense of your overall health and optimal physical functioning, which is something that is a risk for many who follow a vegan diet that has not been carefully thought out.

All the thought and nutritional planning in designing the meals and recipes has been done by myself, a qualified doctor and nutritionist, so that everything is perfectly balanced. There is no calorie counting, tracking or journaling.

The meal plan, advice and recipes in this book are designed to bring simplicity to vegan cooking, providing healthy, balanced meals and snacks that are quick and easy to prepare, delicious *and* weight-loss friendly.

Most vegan recipe books are overly complicated, with endless lists of ingredients and time-consuming recipes. *The Food Effect Diet Vegan* offers straightforward recipes built on healthy ingredients that can be found in any supermarket. There are no obscure ingredients and there is no need to buy expensive foods.

Packaged food labelled 'vegan', or a vegan recipe, is not automatically healthy. Although eating more vegetables, and making recipes incorporating them, definitely has health benefits, a vegan recipe doesn't ensure that it is designed for weight loss. A recipe can easily be vegan-friendly but also extremely high in calories. I have provided a solution to this through *The Food Effect Diet Vegan*, which offers authoritative dietary advice, a structured meal plan and mouth-watering recipes that are simple to prepare, nutritionally balanced, economical and effective for weight loss.

A stress-free diet

The Food Effect Diet Vegan aims to remove any stress around food that being vegan might bring by providing a guidebook that can easily be followed. Alongside the two easy-to-follow stages – the Attack Phase and the Lifestyle Phase with meal plans, options and recipes – this book also provides The Food Effect Tables: an easy reference guide to help you identify which foods are best to eat for weight loss, which you can eat occasionally, and those that you should stay away from.

The recipes are super-simple, demonstrating that preparing healthy vegan food doesn't require you spending hours in the kitchen.

The three keys to diet success

As a self-confessed foodie – as well as a medical doctor with a degree in nutrition – I'm confident in the unique strengths of The Food Effect system, which has already shown proven results. My approach is based on the three key areas of science, choice and taste, which I've channelled into The Food Effect Diet Vegan:

Science – medical and scientific knowledge All the advice in this book is based on a thorough understanding of nutritional science and constant engagement with the latest developments in the world of nutrition, including veganism. It is combined with a comprehensive understanding of health and medical conditions, ensuring that all advice for weight loss addresses nutritional needs for vegans in the most holistic and optimal way.

Choice – tailored solutions I strive to fully appreciate and encompass different lifestyles and eating preferences (for example, cooking at home versus dining out, and so on) so that the advice in this book is workable for everyone. Everything can be tailored to suit your individual needs. In addition to being nutritionally comprehensive for vegans, The Food Effect Diet Vegan advice is simple, practical and realistic, ensuring the optimum chance of success.

Taste – culinary passion and expertise I'm passionate about food and cooking, and I fully appreciate that you want to enjoy your food, so I've channelled this understanding into all my advice to ensure that the meal plans I've provided are both varied and tasty. In addition, I have included useful vegan shopping guides, delicious vegan recipes, and healthy cooking and dining-out advice, which can often be a struggle for vegans. Together, these resources will help you every step along the way, as you discover that a healthy weight-loss diet can be both enjoyable and effective while following a vegan lifestyle.

The combination of science, choice and delicious taste makes this a comprehensive approach to weight loss and improved well-being for all vegans (and those wishing to cut down on animal products and eat more plant-based options). You will become more knowledgeable about healthy eating for a vegan lifestyle in a way that helps you to lead a happier, healthier life – all while looking and feeling fabulous. Best of all, you will achieve all this while still enjoying your food and losing weight. It's a distinctive approach that has shown phenomenal results over the past few years with my growing client base.

How much weight can you lose?

With The Food Effect Diet Vegan you can expect to lose between 6lb and 12lb in the first four weeks alone (during The Food Effect Diet Vegan Attack Phase), and thereafter 1–2lb a week (following The Food Effect Diet Vegan Lifestyle) until you reach your goal weight. The exact amount you can lose will depend on how much weight you have to lose: the more excess weight you're carrying, the more you can expect to lose. Better yet, your new way of eating and The Food Effect Diet Vegan lifestyle will ensure that the weight stays off – so that you get slim and stay slim.

What can you eat?

You'll achieve your goal by eating normal-sized helpings of plant-based proteins, combined with ample healthy carbohydrates and fats. You'll have plenty of fruit and vegetables, with no nonsense telling you that you should cut out fruit because it has too much sugar in it, or that you need to go gluten-free. You will need to cut out certain unhealthy things that you might be eating in excess, but you'll be allowed coffee, carbs, dark chocolate and alcohol from day one. The science behind all this will be explained.

You'll eat three balanced meals a day, as well as two healthy and enjoyable snacks. Everything in the plan is designed so that you won't go hungry. Nothing undermines a weight-loss programme more than the distressing sensation of feeling unsatisfied and hungry – which inevitably ends in bingeing or the need to break the diet. On The Food Effect Diet Vegan you will have a snack mid-afternoon, whether you feel hungry or not. You'll also have a treat every night at whatever time you wish, be it after dinner or at midnight.

If you're the kind of person who 'lives for' bread, pasta and carbs, you won't have to give them up; and if you're the type that can't get through the day without a sugary chocolate bar, sweets or crisps, this plan is going to help you ditch those urges and cravings painlessly for good. It might be challenging for the first day or two, but by cleverly including the right carbohydrates, perfectly designed meals and snacks, and an evening treat, you won't have such a hard time fighting your urges. Within a few days, your cravings will disappear. I can say this with confidence because I've seen it with so many overweight clients, unhealthy eaters and sugar- or junk-food addicts who have succeeded on The Food Effect programme. There's also a whole chapter of tips and tricks for helping you to manage cravings and avoid overeating. The Food Effect Diet Vegan may be new on the shelves, but it has existed for several years – long enough to have helped many clients lose weight with ease, and, thankfully, to keep it off.

Glowing overall health is your aim

Although many vegan diets, cleanses and detoxes will enable you to lose weight, they can leave you with dull, lifeless skin, lacking in energy, and often feeling hungry, tired and even faint. Not only are such diets inadvisable from a health perspective, but they are also unsustainable. In contrast, The Food Effect Diet Vegan recognises that weight loss is just one benefit of healthy eating. When properly planned to include all the key nutrients that can be more challenging for vegans, what we eat has a dramatic impact on how we look, feel and function. A diet should aspire to achieve all of that: weight loss should not come at the expense of overall health and optimal physical functioning.

When it comes to sustainability, the benefit of The Food Effect Diet Vegan lifestyle is that it is self-reinforcing. The more we eat in a wholesome way, the better we look and feel, and the more we want to eat in a wholesome way. Our bodies adapt to an optimum weight, our biological systems improve and we find ourselves full of the energy that lies dormant inside every one of us. You will quite literally *feel* The Food Effect. A diet like this then ceases to be a diet, and instead becomes a fully fledged way of life.

How to develop a healthy eating lifestyle

The three elements involved in developing a healthy eating lifestyle are simplicity, pleasure and sustainability.

Simplicity

Achieving proper nutrition can be confusing for two reasons. The myriad of fad diets, unproven practices and conflicting nutritional information that we are presented with daily in books and magazines, online and on TV can cloud our ability to understand what is (and what is not) good for us. Even some healthy diets are overly complicated due to the inclusion of obscure and overpriced products that are entirely unnecessary for a healthy, balanced diet.

With a thorough understanding of both the human body and the science of nutrition, it is possible to create a vegan diet that is nutritionally complete in accordance with proven science, as well as being simple. I know this is the case, because that is precisely what I have created with The Food Effect Diet Vegan. Simplicity means that the diet is not complicated or expensive, but rather it is made up of ingredients that are available in every local supermarket at reasonable prices. Simplicity also means that putting the diet into practice is not time-consuming – there is no reason why having 'no time' or being 'too busy' should ever be an excuse for unhealthy eating.

Healthy eating should be easily achievable for everyone: from busy parents at home to high-flying corporate executives; for those looking to simply lose weight and feel better, to those with chronic medical conditions who want to improve their symptoms and overall health. The Food Effect programme makes it possible irrespective of your circumstances.

Pleasure

Food is unavoidably a central part of our daily lives. A diet should not be something we go on and come off, but rather it is a way of life. In keeping with this, our food should be delicious and leave us feeling satisfied – not hungry and deprived. The focus of a diet should not only be on what to *exclude*, but more importantly on what to *include*. The elimination of entire food groups, calorie counting and complicated instructions result in eating becoming a chore rather than a pleasure. This inevitably ends with you asking when you can come off the diet and eat all the things you miss again.

Through sensible changes, The Food Effect Diet Vegan will

show you that eating in a healthy, wholesome way is tremendously pleasurable. You will enjoy the textures and tastes found in abundance across all the food groups. You will find yourself enjoying eating and feeling full, and your body will respond in kind – absorbing plenty of nutrients from a variety of sources and becoming slim. To achieve all this is something that appears unachievable in the standard Western diet, yet in reality it's so simple.

Sustainability

It is self-evident that if a diet is going to work and result in a change in our habits, it has to be sustainable, otherwise any benefits achieved will soon be lost. Incorporating all the elements described above – creating a properly designed vegan nutrition plan that keeps things simple and pleasurable – makes lifelong change achievable for everyone.

Once you learn to eat this way, you won't want to go back – it's a change for life.

CHAPTER 1

My Story

From neurosurgeon to nutritionist – and my message to you

OK, I was never a neurosurgeon, but for many years that career was much closer to the path I was travelling than the career I ended up choosing. An ambitious academic child who always wanted to be 'a TV presenter or surgeon' (as expressed in my primary school, thereby gaining many adult laughs), I did in fact pursue my dream of becoming a qualified medical doctor at the prestigious University College London (UCL), much to my dad's delight.

Yet I've also always loved all things to do with health, food and nutrition. I find the science behind it fascinating and am forever challenged and intrigued by what drives us to make certain food choices. Born in sunny South Africa, where healthy eating and good food are a way of life, I've also always had a passion for cooking. My mum is one of the best cooks I know, and I've watched her create the most delicious meals since my childhood (and enjoyed eating them, too). I grew up eating healthy, wholesome, nutritious food without being deprived of anything or given the message that certain foods should be

restricted. Meals were packed with protein, whole-grain carbohydrates, healthy fats (avocados are a staple in South Africa),
fruit and vegetables. I loved salads and everything healthy,
but there was always chocolate in the cupboard and my mum
baked cakes and biscuits regularly.

I was allowed to feel comfortable around food, knowing
that if I wanted to eat a piece of cake as a treat, that was OK
and I wouldn't wake up fat. At the same time, however, I was
shown, in an indirect way, that healthy food was nicer and so
much better for me than unhealthy food and, in fact, I enjoyed
it more. I loved feeling full, satisfied and energised due to
eating hearty, wholesome meals. The chocolate often remained
untouched in the cupboard because I didn't feel that I needed
it. That's what happens when healthy eating becomes a way
of life rather than something restrictive that is associated with
dullness and deprivation, which ultimately leads to cravings
and binges (more on that in Chapter 7).

Thankfully, the balance I was taught from an early age carried me through my teenage years and young adult life, when I
finally decided to hang up the white coat and start my work as
a nutritionist at The Food Effect, my own innovative nutrition
consultancy practice and, later, popular online blog (at www.
thefoodeffect.co.uk). I continue to share my ideas with my
clients and followers today, and I teach people – through the
understanding that healthy eating is actually so much simpler
than we've been led to believe – how to eat better. I'm so grateful to be able to combine my passion for healthy eating with
my knowledge of nutrition and love of exciting new recipes,
in order to create wonderfully delicious (yet simple) meals.
This was a key element in creating The Food Effect Diet, and
I've continued that journey in creating The Food Effect Diet
Vegan. It really is a way of life, and one that I'm excited to be
sharing with you.

How The Food Effect came to be

Despite realising early on that medicine might not be quite the right path for me, I plodded along, spending days (and nights) in hospitals, and ditching sleep in favour of revising for endless exams. During this time, however, I also completed a BSc degree in nutrition at King's College London, which only deepened the chasm between what I was doing and what I felt I should be doing.

More and more, over the course of my last few years as a burnt-out medical student, I realised that I didn't want to spend the rest of my career working as a hospital doctor, but that I still wanted to use the knowledge I had gained from studying medicine and to continue to work in a medically related field, perhaps combining this with my passion for nutrition and the BSc I had gained in it.

Doctors should prescribe healthy foods

I finally had a light-bulb moment during a GP placement in my final year of medicine. That moment came at a point when I had already begun to get extremely frustrated at seeing heart-attack patients who had just had bypass surgery being served fried fish and chips in their hospital beds. I also saw hugely overweight men coming to see their GP, having been newly diagnosed with high blood pressure or high cholesterol (or both), and simply being handed an ongoing prescription for drugs such as statins, without any lifestyle or dietary advice, or even being told to lose weight. I was shocked and appalled.

It angered and frustrated me how little emphasis was put on diet and lifestyle in everyday medical settings. Thankfully, our society is now becoming more aware of the importance of healthy eating, and the fact that doctors often fail to 'prescribe' it is something that's now making headline news. A large number of people are overweight, depressed and diabetic, and have a high risk of heart disease because many doctors fail to provide effective dietary information to their patients. Experts at a 2016 international health conference at the Royal Society of Medicine in London highlighted that the lack of nutritional education available to medical staff amounted to clinical negligence.

Fortunately, I realised this myself back in 2011, and it gave me the impetus I needed to review my career and follow my passion. At the time, I was doing my student placement at a GP practice and was assessing a 15-year-old girl who came in with weakness, exhaustion and shortness of breath. Nothing the doctor had suggested on previous visits had helped her or provided any avenues to explore, and her exhaustion was getting worse and worse. I was given ten minutes alone with the girl to take a brief medical history. I asked her about her menstrual periods, whether she had ever had her iron levels checked and what her current diet was like. In short, this young girl had lost her parents at an early age, lived with her elderly grandmother, who she took care of, and there was no one doing any cooking or food shopping for her. She told me about her very heavy periods and described her daily diet, which consisted of nothing more than white bread or toast, plain white pasta and bags of crisps in between. When I asked her if she ate any fruit or vegetables, or any forms of protein at all, even in the form of baked beans, she told me 'never', the reason being that they were more expensive than her current staples. Even more shocking was the fact that she didn't see anything wrong with this, or realise the importance of those essential basic food groups – not to mention the admission that no doctor had ever asked her about her diet on previous visits. After discussing her diet and nutrition in more detail, it was clear to me that the solution lay in improving it. This episode finally gave me the conviction I needed: expert nutritional advice from a doctor would not just be helpful, but essential in future healthcare. Moreover, I knew I had to build on this idea.

This experience pushed me to take a year out from hospital medicine soon after graduating and do something about my passion for nutrition. Thus The Food Effect nutrition practice was born. In short, my crazy idea, which I planned to do for only a year, went on to become a hugely busy and successful nutrition practice and online blog, all of which I run myself, with my dad – who was initially concerned about my switch from 'neurosurgeon' to nutritionist – now being my guiding rock and greatest supporter. This book has even inspired him to reduce his meat intake and he is now enjoying the vegan recipes.

Starting out

I never dreamed that my little enterprise intended for my year out of clinical practice could become a long-term career. Starting my own business, however, was no easy feat. I had to learn everything from scratch. I'd spent all my years since school either as a medical student or in an NHS hospital, so I had absolutely no idea about anything commercial or business related, but I simply gave it a go and learned along the way.

Although I'll never go back to clinical medicine, I'm grateful that I get to see plenty of interesting cases; often clients come to me who have co-existent medical conditions and are on a range of medications, so my medical knowledge is put to use on a daily basis and was certainly paramount in developing The Food Effect Diet, and The Food Effect Diet Vegan.

All my clients – from day one – have been my motivation, and they are ultimately what led me to write my first book, and now this one. I'm overjoyed when clients report that The Food Effect way of eating has changed their lives on so many levels: improved health, energy, better relationships, looking and feeling better, and loving life more. I am blessed to have the opportunity to help so many people in a field that is so undervalued in our society and healthcare system. And if this book inspires people to find inspiration in vegan eating and living, or to adopt a more plant-based diet, I'd be so grateful too.

What I've learned, and what I'd like to pass on to you

The attributes I developed in becoming a doctor have no doubt helped tremendously in my career as a nutritionist. They include empathy for others, being used to hard work and long hours, and appreciating the importance of patient confidentiality. In addition, everything I learned in my years studying has given me an in-depth knowledge and appreciation for every aspect of the human body, which is hugely beneficial to my career in an area where very few (if any) nutritionists are qualified doctors.

Despite my convictions, I had a hard time for a few months when making the switch. Worrying about what others thought of my decision, and feeling that I had let my parents down, as well as having to explain to everyone I saw or spoke to that I was not carrying on with medicine, was definitely the most challenging aspect of my career transition.

Every cloud, however, has a silver lining, as they say. In my case, the struggle to change career has given me the great advantage of knowing how to motivate people who might otherwise lack the support and encouragement that is required on the journey towards healthy eating and optimal living. The bottom line is: never let the naysayers get in your way, no matter what anyone thinks or however much people try to put you off, whether that's related to your career, diet or lifestyle choices. If I had done so, I'd probably still be stuck in a job that wasn't making me feel good about myself because it simply wasn't the right fit for me. Instead, since leaving medicine, my confidence has soared, and I feel happier and more fulfilled, as you will, too, once you've adopted the lifestyle changes I suggest and start to achieve your health and weight-loss goals. After all, no one should be stuck in a body that doesn't make them feel good – no matter what anyone says.

Give it your best and stay strong

I think being vegan brings additional challenges from what others think and say. Stay strong and remember that you are entitled to eat in a way that makes you feel your best – physically, mentally and emotionally. You do not need to explain yourself to anyone, or apologise for your choices. Be respectful of others and they will be respectful of your choices in return (and if not, don't pay any attention).

Work hard and give everything you do 100 per cent effort, because you only get out what you put in. My message to you is that you should go for it and work hard. If you never try, you'll never know. This applies to everything, from work and business, to healthy eating and living.

Confidence also plays a huge role in the success of any pursuit; you don't need to be perfect, but if you believe you can do something, you will succeed. Start this book with a positive outlook and throw any negative thoughts out the window! There's no place for 'I can't do this' or 'It won't work for me because of xyz ...' If you make excuses, there'll always be a reason why now is not the right time. That's a key message of The Food Effect Diet Vegan: don't settle for an unhappy, mediocre version of yourself when you can look and feel the best you can be.

If you face mental or emotional obstacles when embarking on this new way of life, hopefully the words of the famous quote from Marianne Williamson's book *A Return to Love* will inspire you:

'Our deepest fear is not that we are inadequate. Our deepest fear is that we are powerful beyond measure. It is our light, not our darkness that most frightens us. We ask ourselves, "Who am I to be brilliant, gorgeous, talented and fabulous?" Actually, who are you not to be?'

Who are you not to be brilliant, gorgeous, talented and fabulous – in a body that you feel amazing in, eating in a way that makes you happy? Yes, there are those who might try to put you off, but remember that their attitude might be born out of a fear of their own inability to change and uncertainty as to the potential that lies within you. However, just imagine the positive knock-on effects of embarking on such life-enhancing changes, for those around you, as well as yourself. The possibilities really are endless.

Thus, with some little personal anecdotes from me, a whole host of reasons for joining the journey that you simply cannot refute, and a tiny taster of what this exciting new lifestyle has in store for you, you're now ready to move on to Chapter 2, which is all about getting started and understanding The Food Effect Diet Vegan.

CHAPTER 2

Getting Started

Understanding The Food Effect Diet Vegan

With so much to gain, it's understandable that by now you're probably eager to begin The Food Effect Diet Vegan, in order to experience The Food Effect for yourself. By doing so, you will begin a journey that will not only help you to lose weight but will also enhance your overall health, vitality and longevity.

The first step is to follow Phase 1, the 28-day Food Effect Diet Vegan Attack Phase, before moving on to the next phase, The Food Effect Diet Vegan Lifestyle. These are discussed further in this chapter, and in a lot more detail that includes the meal options and plans laid out in full in Chapters 11 and 12.

Before you start the programme, you need some basic information on what to eat – and what to avoid. I provide this later in this chapter in The Food Effect Tables, which illustrate the effects of different foods on health and weight. You will also find the key guidelines in this chapter, laid out in my rules and tips for healthy eating and weight loss.

Chapters 3 to 10 provide you with the essential knowledge you will need to understand the rationale behind The Food Effect approach. Knowledge is power, as the saying goes, so don't skip these sections. They also provide a wealth of tips and tricks on everything from dining out healthily and drinking alcohol to snacking smartly and banishing cravings – all while following a vegan lifestyle.

Chapters 3, 4 and 6 provide valuable information about carbohydrates, protein and fats: which ones you're going to be eating, and what you'll be avoiding and why.

Once you begin this programme, you will never look at food and eating in the same way again. You will still enjoy food and will love to eat, but you will do so with an appreciation and understanding that you probably didn't have before. There will be no more hunger or deprivation, and no more fad diets. The Food Effect Diet Vegan is about finally learning how to lose weight while eating a well-balanced vegan diet for the rest of your life.

This chapter outlines the foods you can and can't eat. It couldn't be easier.

What is veganism?

Veganism is not a diet but a lifestyle that avoids all animal products, including meat, fish, eggs and dairy, and any food products derived from animals, such as honey and Worcestershire sauce.

Following a healthy balanced vegan diet, such as The Food Effect Diet Vegan, can bring great health benefits, including increased energy and metabolic rate (thanks to all the plant-based fibre), and clearer, more youthful-looking skin (thanks to all the vitamins, minerals and antioxidants).

When following a vegan diet, it's important to eat a wide range of foods in order to obtain sufficient nutrients, such as protein, omega-3 fatty acids and vitamin B12, that ▶

are found in abundance in animal sources but are less available in plant-based sources. The Food Effect Diet Vegan includes an abundance of fruits and vegetables, beans and legumes, wholegrains, healthy carbohydrates, plant-based proteins, nuts and seeds, and dairy alternatives, to ensure all your nutritional needs are met.

The 'Eat this', 'Be careful' and 'Stay away' tables

In this section you will find all the food groups (fruit, vegetables, legumes, fats and oils, nuts and seeds, grains and carbohydrates, proteins, dairy alternatives, beverages and condiments) laid out in tables, divided into 'Eat this', 'Be careful' and 'Stay away' columns to make knowing what to eat and what to avoid simple and effortless. Once you've looked at the tables a few times, you probably won't need to look back at them often. As I've stressed, The Food Effect Diet Vegan way of eating becomes a lifestyle rather than a diet.

The titles at the tops of the columns are pretty self-explanatory, and although I wouldn't advocate that you never have a piece of cake again (after all, what's a birthday without some cake?), as a general rule 'Stay away' means exactly that, as all the foods listed under this column do absolutely nothing to benefit your health, and will just prevent you from achieving your weight-loss goals. 'Be careful' might mean 'consume in moderation', as in the case of vegan mayonnaise or maple syrup, or alternatively that a food is not the best option but is not 'terrible', (for example, white rice, white potatoes and white pasta), so you can have them occasionally, if that's all that's available; for example, when dining out at a restaurant.

By eating The Food Effect Diet Vegan way, made easy with these tables, you'll get healthy and lose weight – about 6–12lb in the first four weeks alone (during the Attack Phase), and thereafter 1–2lb a week (following the Lifestyle Phase), until you reach your goal weight. (As mentioned earlier, the exact amount of weight you lose will vary according to how much you need to lose: the more excess weight you're carrying, the more you can expect to lose.) Better yet, your new way of eating and The Food Effect Diet Vegan Lifestyle will ensure that the weight stays off – so, as well as getting slim, you'll stay slim.

When cooking at home, you should always aim to keep to the foods in the 'Eat this' column – such as brown rice and whole-wheat, chickpea or red-lentil pasta – and these are the foods that are included in the suggested meal options. They are beneficial to both your overall health and weight-loss goals. For most of the carbohydrates and proteins, as well as fruit, portions are specified in the meal options in both the Attack and Lifestyle Phases. Most vegetables (such as spinach, tomatoes and cucumber) can be eaten freely with your meals, and if portions are not specified, it means that this is the case.

Anything with an asterisk (*) denotes a healthy food (that is, an 'Eat this' food) that need not be avoided but should be consumed in moderation due to its calorie content.

Fruit

EAT THIS	BE CAREFUL	STAY AWAY
All fresh fruit	Dried fruit with added sugar	Bananas
Dried fruit (no added sugar)*	Tinned fruit in sugar/syrup	Fruit cakes/crumbles
Tinned fruit in natural juices (no added sugar)		Fruit juice
		Fruit pies/pastries

Vegetables

EAT THIS	BE CAREFUL	STAY AWAY
All the following (fresh/ frozen/tinned in water)		
Artichoke	White potato	
Asparagus		
Aubergine		
Avocado*		
Baby corn		
Beansprouts		
Beetroot		
Broccoli		
Brussels sprouts		
Butternut squash		
Cabbage		
Carrot		
Cauliflower		
Celeriac		
Celery		

EAT THIS	BE CAREFUL	STAY AWAY
Chives		
Corn		
Courgette		
Cucumber		
Fennel		
Garlic		
Green beans		
Hearts of palm		
Jicama		
Kale		
Kohlrabi		
Leek		
Lettuce (all varieties)		
Mangetout		
Mushroom		
Okra		
Onion		
Pak choi		

EAT THIS	BE CAREFUL	STAY AWAY
Parsley		
Parsnip		
Pepper		
Radish		
Rocket		
Spinach		
Spring onion		
Sweet potato		
Tomato		
Turnip		
Watercress		

Legumes

EAT THIS	BE CAREFUL	STAY AWAY
All the following (dried/ frozen/tinned in water)		
Black beans	Baked beans	
Butter beans		
Cannellini beans		

EAT THIS	BE CAREFUL	STAY AWAY
Chickpeas		
Fava beans		
Kidney beans		
Lentils		
Peas		
Chickpea pasta		
Red lentil pasta		

Fats and oils

EAT THIS	BE CAREFUL	STAY AWAY
Avocado*	Vegan mayonnaise	Hydrogenated vegetable oils
Avocado oil*		
Canola oil*	Non-stick cooking sprays	Palm oil
Coconut oil*	Groundnut/peanut oil	Shortening
Flaxseed oil*	Reduced-fat vegan margarine, trans-fat free	Vegan margarine
Guacamole* (home-made)		Vegetable oil
Hummus* (home-made/ reduced fat)		
Natural nut butters*		

EAT THIS	BE CAREFUL	STAY AWAY
Nuts* (see 'Nuts and seeds')		
Olive oil*		
Olives*		
Rapeseed oil*		
Sunflower oil*		
Sesame oil*		
Tahini*		

Nuts and seeds

EAT THIS	BE CAREFUL	STAY AWAY
Almonds*	Salted nuts	Caramelised nuts
Brazil nuts*		
Cashew nuts*		
Chia seeds		
Linseed/flaxseed		
Nut butters*		
Peanuts*		
Pecan nuts*		

EAT THIS	BE CAREFUL	STAY AWAY
Poppy seeds*		
Pumpkin seeds*		
Sesame seeds*		
Sunflower seeds*		
Walnuts*		

Grains and carbohydrates

EAT THIS	BE CAREFUL	STAY AWAY
Barley	Air-popped/low-fat popcorn	Caramelised popcorn
Brown rice	Fruit chutney	Crisps
Brown rice cakes	Jam	Dairy-free chocolate spread
Bulgur wheat	Low-fat (store-bought) vegan bran/healthy muffins	French fries/chips
Corn	Low-fat refined (white flour) crackers	Fried noodles
Dark chocolate* (dairy free)	Agave syrup	Fried rice
Home-made healthy vegan muffin/treat* (see page 221 and recipes for 'Snacks and sweet treats'	Maple syrup	High-fat crackers (e.g. Snackers)
Kasha	Matzo crackers	High-fat granola
Oats, oatmeal, porridge	Molasses	Muffins (vegan, store-bought)

EAT THIS	BE CAREFUL	STAY AWAY
Polenta	Muesli mixes (no added sugar)	Packaged waffles
Quinoa	Oatcakes	Refined high-sugar breakfast cereals
Rye	Pretzels	Refined sugar (all varieties)
Rye bread	White bread, bagels, pitta	Store-bought/bakery vegan cakes
Rye crackers	White pasta	Sweets (hard and jelly) made with refined sugar
Spelt	White rice	Tarts
Sourdough bread		
Sweet potatoes	White tortilla wraps	Vegan biscuits made with refined sugar
Wholemeal/ multigrain bread	Whole-grain breakfast cereals	Vegan croissants
Whole-wheat bagels, pitta		Vegan cupcakes
Whole-wheat couscous		Vegan doughnuts
Whole-wheat low-fat crackers		Vegan pastries
Whole-wheat pasta		Vegan pies/pie crust
Wild rice		
Brown rice pasta		
Chickpea pasta		
Red lentil pasta		

Proteins

EAT THIS	BE CAREFUL	STAY AWAY
Beans (see 'Legumes' above		Dairy-free coffee creamers
Chickpeas	Dairy-free frozen yoghurt (FroYo)	Deep-fried tofu
Lentils	Dairy-free yoghurts (soya) with added sugar (e.g. Alpro fruit flavours)	Fried falafel balls
Edamame beans		Fried vegan meat substitutes
Tofu (steamed, baked, grilled, sautéed with minimal oil)	Soya milk (with added sugar)	Full-fat dairy-free yoghurts with added sugar
Miso soup		
Jackfruit (canned in water)		
Non-GMO soya and soya products (natural ingredients)		Full-fat vegan cream cheese made from coconut/soya oil
Hummus*		Non-dairy artificial cream substitutes (e.g. Rich's Whip)
Vegan burgers (e.g. Beyond Burger, Fry's brand, or homemade)		Vegan pies
Almond- or cashew-based non-dairy cream cheese (e.g. Nush foods)		Yellow/hard processed vegan cheeses made from coconut/soya oil
Tempeh		
Low-fat plant-based milks and dairy substitute products (see 'Dairy alternatives' below)		

EAT THIS	BE CAREFUL	STAY AWAY
Nut butters* (see 'Nuts and seeds' above)		
Nuts* (see 'Nuts and seeds' above)		
Unsweetened soya yoghurts		
Unsweetened soya milk		
Baked falafel balls (or health-store bought)		
Vegan protein powder (flavoured with sweetener, no refined sugar)		

Dairy alternatives

EAT THIS	BE CAREFUL	STAY AWAY
Unsweetened almond milk	Coconut cream (full fat)	Coconut yoghurt with added sugar
Unsweetened oat milk	Dairy-free frozen yoghurt	Dairy-free coffee creamers (made from artificial ingredients)
Unsweetened rice milk	Dairy-free yoghurts (soya) with added sugar (e.g. Alpro fruit flavours)	Full-fat vegan cream cheese made from coconut/soya oil
Unsweetened soya milk	Plant-based milks (e.g. almond, cashew, coconut) with added sugar	Non-dairy cream substitutes (made from artificial ingredients)
Unsweetened hemp milk		
Unsweetened light coconut milk		

EAT THIS	BE CAREFUL	STAY AWAY
Unsweetened cashew milk		
Almond- or cashew-based non-dairy cream cheese (e.g. Nush foods or Kite Hill)		Yellow/hard processed vegan cheeses made from coconut oil
Unsweetened soya yoghurt (e.g. Alpro)		
Coconut water	Unsweetened coconut yoghurt	Vegan margarine
Vegan protein powder (flavoured with sweetener, no refined sugar)		

Beverages

DRINK THIS	BE CAREFUL	STAY AWAY
Bloody Mary*	Beer	Alcopops
Champagne*	Hot cocoa (low sugar)	Amaretto sour
Coffee*	Mimosa	Cocktails mixed with energy drinks
Gin and diet tonic*	Mojito	Cocktails with cola mixers
Vodka and diet tonic*		
Green tea	Pina colada	Energy drinks

DRINK THIS	BE CAREFUL	STAY AWAY
Herbal tea	Rum and Diet Coke	Frozen daiquiri
Red wine*	Sweetened plant-based milks	Fruit juice with or without added sugar
Red/white wine spritzer*	Vodka cranberry	Hot chocolate (with added sugar)
Tea, regular		Malibu and Coke/fruit juice
Vodka and soda water (with lemon/lime)*		Margarita
Water, sparkling mineral water		Dairy-free creamy liqueurs
White wine*		Rum and Coke
		Soft drinks, including diet sodas
Unsweetened almond/plant-based milks		
Whisky*		
Tequila*		
Coconut water		
Martini*		

Condiments, spreads and sweeteners

EAT THIS	BE CAREFUL	STAY AWAY
All herbs and spices	Agave syrup	Dairy-free chocolate spread
Chilli sauce (without oil)	Fruit chutneys	Full-fat bottled salad dressings

EAT THIS	BE CAREFUL	STAY AWAY
Cinnamon	Hoisin sauce	High-fructose corn syrup
Hummus*		
Ketchup (reduced sugar and salt)	HP sauce	Refined sugar
Lemon juice	Jam	Vegan margarine
Marmite	Maple syrup	
Mustard	Molasses	
Salsa	Soy sauce (not low sodium)	
Soy sauce (reduced sodium)		
Sriracha (hot sauce)	Sweet chilli sauce	
Sweeteners including stevia and xylitol		
Vinegars (all varieties)	Vegan mayonnaise	

The fundamental principles

These following principles underpin The Food Effect Diet Vegan. Following them will make losing weight achievable, as well as ensuring that maintaining a healthy weight will not be a lifetime struggle.

Eat whole, natural foods Avoid packaged, processed foods as much as possible. This means eating whole, natural foods that are close to, if not in, their natural state. For example: fresh fruit, vegetables, whole grains, nuts, seeds, beans, chickpeas and lentils. The shorter the list of ingredients on a package of food, the better it is. Nowadays there is an ever-increasing amount of vegan snacks, treats, cheeses and ready meals becoming available. Although this is great, they are not always healthy, so check labels and don't be fooled by a label just because it states 'vegan'.

Make sure you never get too hungry Long gaps between meals disrupt your blood-sugar levels, leading to excessive hunger, cravings and, often, stress eating. The outcome is that when you do eventually eat, you're so hungry that it takes a lot more food to feel satisfied, and it's unlikely that you'll binge on celery sticks or apples. Eating small, healthy snacks between meals will help keep your blood sugar stable and your metabolism going strong. The suggested snacks in the meal options will guide you.

Stay well hydrated Often, when we think that we're hungry, we're actually just thirsty. Water aids weight loss by keeping your cells functioning at their fat-burning best, and it also helps your kidneys to flush out the excess toxins and chemicals, which might be slowing down your metabolism. Make sure that you drink plenty of water throughout the day, as well as one to two glasses before every meal or snack you have. See more about this in The Food Effect Rules.

Slow down your eating and enjoy your food Focus on the food you're eating and don't wolf it down. Avoid eating dinner in front of the TV or lunch in front of your computer. Take time out to enjoy your meal, and pay attention to what you're eating. This will ensure that your brain registers when you've eaten enough food, before it's too late.

Eat healthy fats – don't go fat-free This means eating good, healthy unsaturated fats found in nuts, peanut butter, avocados, olive oil and various other healthy oils. Incorporating good fats into your diet will help to reduce sugar cravings, increase energy levels and keep you fuller for longer. Whereas too much fat can cause weight gain, too little of the right fats prevents your cells from functioning properly, which affects fat metabolism, hormone balance and energy – all leading to weight gain. There's more detailed information on fats in Chapter 6.

Don't shun carbs Instead, stick to whole-grain, unrefined carbohydrates such as oats, wholemeal or rye bread, brown rice, sweet potatoes and quinoa. Slow-release carbs from whole-grain sources will give you the get-up-and-go you need to stay active and full of energy while keeping your metabolism going strong and steady all day (and night). They are also great sources of fibre and various other essential nutrients, such as the B vitamins niacin, thiamine and folate, and minerals, such as zinc, iron, magnesium and manganese.

Know yourself and be realistic Each of us has different needs, goals and preferences, combined with a different body type and genetic make-up. You have to recognise your individual needs and be realistic about the changes you can make; for example, if you enjoy having your evening snack late at night, there's no point in trying to force yourself to eat it earlier in the day. Evidence has refuted the myth that calories eaten late at night are worse, and has proven that a calorie is a calorie is a calorie. Whether you eat it at 7pm or midnight, there's no difference weight-wise; it's your overall daily consumption that counts, which is why you're allowed an evening snack every night.

Eat a rainbow Whether they are fresh, frozen or tinned – try to increase and vary your intake of fruit and vegetables, which, thankfully, being vegan definitely encourages. You'll feel so much better and your body will benefit from all the added vitamins, nutrients, antioxidants and fibre. Diets rich in fruit and vegetables have been proven to decrease the risk of heart attacks, strokes and a variety of cancers, and healthy, glowing skin is another by-product of eating a colourful, varied diet.

Know your portions Just because it's healthy and vegan, it doesn't mean that it can't make you gain weight. This is a common misconception when people adopt a vegan diet. Even if you stick to healthy foods, you still have to watch your portion sizes and quantities when consuming foods such as nuts, hummus, avocado, olive oil and dark chocolate (in other words, all the things marked with an asterisk in The Food Effect Tables). They might be healthy, but that does not mean that you can eat them freely. There's definitely a benefit in consuming a little olive oil, but pouring it liberally over your pasta, and dipping your bread in it, will lead to excessive calories and weight gain. The same goes for nuts – learn what a normal serving size looks like (it's very easy to eat a whole big bag) and limit yourself to that (see page 101 for portion sizes).

The Food Effect Diet Vegan Rules

These rules go hand in hand with the above principles for healthy eating and weight loss. If you follow both sets of guidelines, you'll be guaranteed weight-loss success, and you will look and feel better than ever. The Food Effect Diet Vegan diet is all about being the best version of you – so there are no excuses for not following these rules.

1. **Prepare, prepare, prepare** This is the golden rule of healthy eating habits. The more organised you are, the easier, and more likely, healthy eating and living will be. Make your own lunch, where possible; pre-chop vegetables to have on hand for meals and snacks; and keep your fridge and cupboards stocked with the right healthy foods.

2. **Avoid highly processed and packaged foods as much as possible** Read the labels on food products – don't buy what you can't pronounce or have never heard of. As mentioned earlier, something labelled vegan does *not* mean it's healthy.

3. **Don't go hungry** Always carry healthy snacks with you if you know you're going to be out and about for a while or working long hours. For convenience, all snacks are listed daily in your plan, and there is also a long list of options in Chapter 12, so there's really no excuse. But...

4. **Don't graze** Eating regularly doesn't mean that you should be constantly picking throughout the day. A few nuts here and there do add up. Stick to your three meals and two snacks per day – and nothing outside that. Have them whenever you feel it suits you best to do so.

5. **Ditch the white stuff** Cutting out the white stuff (white sugar, white bread, flour, pasta and sugary, low-fibre cereals – not almond milk and cauliflower) is one of the easiest ways to lose weight and improve your health. Most processed, refined carbohydrate foods are just empty calories with little fibre and goodness.

6. **Don't cut out all starchy foods** As I will explain in Chapter 3, this is a recipe for long-term diet disaster.

7. **Eat good fats** As I will explain in more detail in Chapter 6, you need some good fat in order to burn fat. This means eating good, healthy unsaturated fats found in nuts, peanut butter, avocados, olive oil and various other healthy oils, as mentioned in the Principles above. These are all included (in specified amounts) in the plan, as they are proven to lower the risk of heart disease and aid the body in the absorption of vitamins and minerals, as well as helping with satiety, cravings and weight loss.

8. **Avoid trans fats** Often listed under the names 'hydrogenated oil' or 'hydrogenated vegetable fat', and found in many processed vegan-friendly foods, these fats are toxic

and have no health benefits whatsoever. Be aware that manufacturers don't have to note them on labels if they are below 0.5g, but this can mount up.

9. **Eat vegetables and fruit** You can eat as much salad, and fresh, steamed, stir-fried and baked vegetables as you like (within the specified meals), as long as they don't have added dressing or oil (apart from the amount specified in the plan). You can add as much lemon juice, balsamic vinegar or apple cider vinegar, as well as seasonings (salt and pepper) and spices, as you like. Fruit is also included in healthy, specified portions in the plan.

10. **Eat slowly and chew thoroughly** Take time to enjoy and savour all your food (meals and snacks). Chewing your food properly will aid efficient digestion, stop you from overeating and reduce any uncomfortable bloating that you might experience from eating too quickly.

11. **Drink plenty of water** As explained in the Principles section above, make sure you drink one to two glasses of water before every meal or snack you have to keep yourself hydrated. If you have difficulty drinking enough plain water (around 2 litres a day), herbal teas, green tea (hot or iced) or lemon in hot water are all just as good.

12. **No sugary soft drinks or fruit juice** The reason for this is explained in Chapter 3.

13. **Weigh yourself** Weigh yourself first thing in the morning, after you've gone to the toilet to empty your bladder, without any clothes on. In the Attack Phase I'll be advising you to weigh yourself every day, for the first four weeks. The theory behind this, and why it is beneficial for weight loss, is explained in Chapter 11, which introduces you to Phase 1

and starting the Attack Phase. After the first four weeks, once you're at the Lifestyle Phase, you should weigh yourself in the same way, once a week.

14. **Start your morning with a mug of warm water and apple cider vinegar** It's even better than warm water and lemon – often promoted as the healthiest way to start the day – so my advice is to kick off the morning with a mug of warm water and apple cider vinegar. Put a tablespoon of apple cider vinegar – a wonder food with lots of healing properties – into a mug of warm water. Drinking this will hydrate you and cleanse your digestive system. It's more effective than a probiotic, and is the perfect way to set up your body for its daily food intake ahead, as well as helping to prevent bloating. Even though it's vinegar it actually neutralises acid and puts your body in a good pH balance so that your internal systems work well. It can also kill bad bacteria in the stomach and intestine, and promotes good gut bacteria. I must admit that I personally struggle with the taste 'straight up' so I add a teaspoon or two of stevia or agave syrup to make it more palatable. There's absolutely no health downside to doing this, so do try it.

15. **Have a big hot drink with your breakfast (and midmorning)** This provides a warm, comforting start to the day that, combined with a good breakfast, leaves you feeling satisfied for the day ahead. It can be tea, coffee, a herbal or green tea. You can add almond or any plant-based milk with no added sugar. Sweeteners such as stevia and xylitol are allowed with no restriction (see Chapter 3).

16. **A word on caffeine** Although excess caffeine is obviously not good, caffeine from good-quality coffee (without added sugar or syrups) is packed full of antioxidants and has been shown to have tremendous health benefits. When consumed before

a workout, it has also been shown to boost performance and stamina while exercising. Stick to a maximum of two coffees a day, preferably early in the day – not late in the afternoon or the evening, so as not to disrupt your sleep.

17. **Limit (but don't shun) alcohol** There are many health benefits to alcohol as long as it's consumed in moderation, and you stick to the right choices. Drink no more than three glasses a week during the Attack Phase, and a maximum of one per night (up to seven drinks a week) once on the Lifestyle Phase. Keep to the drinks listed under 'Drink this' in the table (on page 36), although it's fine to drink those in the 'Be careful' category occasionally. Sticking to this limit will help you to lose weight, clear your head and improve your energy levels, without making you cut out alcohol completely. For more on alcohol, see Chapter 9.

18. **Don't give up or get despondent** We're all human and have our ups and downs. Although you are aiming to be disciplined in your food choices, The Food Effect Diet Vegan healthy-eating lifestyle is not intended to starve or deprive you. If you do slip up, it's certainly not the end of the world. Don't feel as though you've failed and then set yourself back further by going on a total binge fest – just accept it and move on.

Enjoy your Food Effect journey and remember that as long as you continue to be consistent in the process, you will reap the benefits and get fantastic results.

The more stringent rules specific to the Attack Phase (the first 28 days) are laid out in Chapter 11. Both phases of The Food Effect Diet Vegan (all meal and snack options) are based on the foods in the tables in this chapter, incorporating mainly 'Eat this' foods, and avoiding anything from the 'Stay away' list.

CHAPTER 3

Don't Shun Carbohydrates

Dispelling the myths

In today's dieting age, carbohydrates – or carbs as they're commonly known – are often seen as the enemy, associated with piling on the pounds and increasing body fat. In reality, nothing could be further from the truth. Carbohydrates can actually help you to reach your weight-loss goals – you just need to know which ones to eat, and which ones to avoid.

You might think that no one who is vegan would ever try to cut out carbs, as they commonly form a large part of most vegan diets (and healthy carbs are a rich source of nutrients essential for vegans), but I've seen many popular vegan influencers on Instagram and YouTube promoting their 'low carb vegan diet' and the sad reality is that many people think that they should be following this in an attempt to lose weight.

Of course, a healthy diet is the key to losing weight, but for some reason the first thing people often think they need to do is stop eating carbs, and sadly this false message has become prevalent in the vegan community too. Cutting out carbs might lead to weight loss at first, but it won't be sustainable, and you'll end up tired, lethargic, cranky and irritable. You will also pile on the pounds the minute you start eating normally again – because living off tofu, lettuce leaves and steamed broccoli is not sustainable for the rest of your life.

The fact is that cutting out carbs can slow down your metabolism and the process of fat burning, preventing you from reaching your goal weight, because your body needs carbs to function properly (more on this later). Without carbs, your body will actually hold on to excess fat because it's lacking its main energy supply. Cutting out all starchy foods is therefore a major diet disaster; however, when eating them, you must stick to the right ones. These include whole-grain unrefined carbohydrates such as wholemeal or rye bread, quinoa, whole-wheat, brown rice or chickpea pasta, brown rice, sweet potatoes and oats (everything listed under the 'Eat this' column for carbohydrates in the tables on page 32). These are great sources of fibre and full of a variety of other nutrients.

Although it's widely accepted that highly processed refined carbohydrates (those listed under the 'Stay away' column in the same table) are bad for health and can contribute to weight gain, whole-grain complex carbohydrates are actually full of fibre and various other essential nutrients, which help to keep you fuller for longer by regulating your appetite – the key to successful sustainable weight loss. The nutrients in wholegrain carbs are especially important for vegans – (for example, brown rice is rich in B vitamins), who might not be getting these from other sources.

Before getting on to practical aspects, such as guiding you on portion sizes to enable you to lose weight without cutting out carbs, here is some basic nutritional information to help you understand The Food Effect approach to carbohydrates.

What are carbohydrates?

Carbohydrates are our brain and body's main source of energy, which we all need in order to carry out everyday activities. Through my experience with countless clients, friends and

s both a doctor and a nutritionist, I've seen the harm
ing out carbs can do to people, in both the short and
m. Insufficient carbohydrate consumption can cause the
ng problems:

Temporary unsustainable weight loss

When you reduce your carbohydrate intake, you may notice how quickly – as if by magic – the weight falls off. But it's not fat you're losing – it's water. When carbs are stored in the body in the form of glycogen, each gram of carbohydrate stores three to four times its weight in water, so as soon as you cut carbs and start using your glycogen stores you'll lose a fair amount of water weight. This is particularly the case if you're on a high-protein diet that depletes your glycogen stores. Although everyone loves seeing the number on the scale go down and this might give you a great boost, you will soon plateau once you've lost the extra water weight and your body clings on to its fat stores, as it's being depleted of its main energy source: carbohydrates. Once your body realises there's a food shortage, it goes into starvation mode – again, something I've seen with many clients who've come to me having cut out carbs, yet remained overweight. Your metabolism automatically begins to slow down in order to expend as little energy as possible. You will also be tired and irritable (as explained below), and, as a result, you will lose any motivation to stick to such unrealistic weight-loss plans. The outcome is that the weight loss will taper off and you will stop losing weight entirely. Moreover, when you do begin eating carbs again (because such plans are unsustainable in the long term), you will pile on the pounds even more than normal, as your whole metabolism and ability to burn carbs will have slowed down.

Muscle cramps and low energy levels

Anyone who carries out physical exercise will need to replenish glycogen stores that are depleted during exercise, making carbohydrate consumption essential – especially post-workout. Carbohydrates are the body's main source of energy for fuelling all exercise, including cardio and resistance training. Cut out carbs and your energy levels will drop. The result of decreased levels of your body's stored carbohydrates (glycogen) is a decreased ability to produce power, and poorer workouts mean poorer results. Whole-grain carbohydrates are an important source of iron, magnesium and B vitamins, all of which are critical in maintaining energy levels and muscle function. Many people are already deficient in magnesium, so without a healthy supply of the right carbs, all your cells slow down and your muscles suffer as a result.

Fatigue and poor mental function

Carbs are not only the body's main source of energy, but also the brain's. When you cut out carbs, the brain is essentially running on empty – especially once glycogen levels are low and become depleted. Once all the glycogen is gone, your body breaks down fat and runs off carbon compounds called ketones. This results in a dry mouth, bad breath, weakness, tiredness, dizziness, nausea and brain fog – you might even feel as though you have flu. Eventually, your body adapts to running on ketones so you get used to it, but you certainly won't be functioning at your best, as this isn't the body's preferred fuel source. Carbohydrates also play a major role in maintaining hormone balance, which is vital for sufficient and optimal bodily function.

Cravings

If your blood-sugar levels are irregular (which can be a result of either insufficient carbohydrate consumption or eating the wrong carbs), you are more likely to crave bad foods. The key is not to avoid carbs, but to make sure you consume the right ones.

The tables in Chapter 2 are a good guide as to which carbs will help you achieve your goals. Contrary to popular belief, carbohydrates are also what muscles want and need for optimum functioning – they are what refuels them. When we don't replenish our stores (by cutting carbs out when dieting, for example), our bodies produce hunger hormones to encourage us to seek them out. Our body will do whatever it takes to let us know it needs food. Hunger, deprivation and cravings are certainly not the ideal basis for weight-loss success.

Constipation

Whole-grain carbohydrate intake (what The Food Effect lifestyle promotes) is a major factor in how much fibre you consume. Fibre, found in whole grains, fruit and vegetables (see the 'Eat this' column on the table on pages 26–33), not only helps to stabilise blood-sugar levels, thereby preventing hunger and cravings, and reducing the risk of obesity and chronic diseases such as diabetes and bowel cancer, but it also helps to keep your bowel habits regular.

Moodiness

When you cut out healthy carbohydrates, fruit and whole grains, your mental health and happiness go right along with them. This is not solely because you're living off tofu and lettuce leaves, but because carbohydrates, including whole-grain unrefined carbs, increase the brain's level of the feel-good hormone serotonin.

The different types of carbohydrate

Carbohydrates can be divided into two main types: simple (sugars) and complex (starch and fibre). The difference between the two lies in their molecular structure. Simple carbohydrates have a simple molecular structure and complex carbs have a more complex one. This affects how they're broken down and absorbed by our bodies.

Simple carbohydrates

Simple carbohydrates are made up of one to two sugar molecules and are broken down and digested very quickly due to their simple structure. Examples of foods containing these carbs are sweets, cakes, biscuits, sugary drinks and sodas, white bread and white rice. When consumed, these foods are rapidly converted to sugars, which are directly absorbed in the blood in the form of glucose, leading to rapidly elevated blood-sugar levels. The glucose provides instant energy, but if not burned or used up (which it rarely is, unless these foods are consumed right before a workout), they are converted to, and stored as, fat – leading to weight gain and potentially other health issues (see page 54). It's for this reason that these foods are placed in the 'Stay away' or, at best, 'Be careful' categories in the tables in Chapter 2.

Complex carbohydrates

The longer chains of sugar molecules in complex carbohydrates, compared to those in simple carbs, take longer to break down in the gut, requiring more time for digestion. This slows down the breakdown process and supplies the body with sustained energy and increased satiety for a longer period of time. Examples of complex carbohydrates are brown rice, sweet potatoes, rolled oats and wholemeal bread. Since these carbohydrates require more time to be broken down, they are constantly used up by the body and are not immediately converted to, or stored as, fat (unless eaten in large amounts, which is why portion sizes are specified in the meal options).

The glycaemic index

The glycaemic index (GI) is a ranking of carbohydrates from 0 to 100, according to how quickly they raise blood-sugar levels after they are eaten. As discussed earlier, simple carbohydrates raise blood sugar rapidly, and therefore have a high GI, whereas complex carbohydrates take longer to break down in the body, and thus have a lower GI, indicating that they don't cause a spike in blood-sugar levels. For this reason, these are always preferable.

A note on sourdough bread

Although sourdough bread might look similar to regular white bread, it's been shown to have a lower glycaemic index (GI) and therefore a much better effect on blood sugar and insulin levels than other types of bread.

Researchers believe that the sourdough fermentation process modifies the structure of the carbohydrate molecules. This reduces the bread's GI and slows down the speed at which sugars enter the bloodstream. Sourdough bread contains higher levels of folate and antioxidants than other breads, and its lower phytate levels allow your body to absorb the nutrients it contains more easily, making it one of the healthiest choices for vegans (and non-vegans). Additionally, the fermentation process alters the structure of the gluten, making sourdough much easier to digest than other breads, especially for those who don't tolerate gluten well. Sourdough bread contains lower amounts of gluten and its prebiotic- and probiotic-like properties might help improve digestion. It's for this reason that it's included under the 'Eat this' column along with wholemeal and rye bread.

Low-GI carbs

Extremely nutritious due to the abundance of vitamins, minerals and fibre they contain, the low-GI carbs are the carbohydrates that are included in The Food Effect Diet Vegan meal plan and options. Because fibre cannot be digested by the body, it slows down the digestion of the digestible carbs, so blood-sugar levels do not spike, thereby promoting satiety and helping to manage cravings. Low-GI carbs (such as the complex carbohydrates mentioned previously) provide steady energy levels, which are extremely beneficial throughout the day, including after exercise.

Sweet potatoes, for example, have a lower GI than white potatoes, as they take longer to break down into sugar in the body. Sweet potatoes are therefore the healthier choice compared with white potatoes, and certainly a wiser option for people who have diabetes or who are managing high blood-sugar levels. Additionally, sweet potatoes are richer in the antioxidant beta-carotene, which helps to defend against cellular damage which can lead to cancer, heart disease and skin ageing. And apart from being super-healthy, they're super-tasty. You'll see a lot of sweet potatoes in The Food Effect Diet Vegan meal options, so you won't feel deprived of delicious carbs. You can enjoy them mashed or baked whole or in wedges. They're also delicious in a vegan stew, chilli or tagine (see the recipes in Chapter 13). If you're not a sweet potato lover already, your taste buds will soon get used to them, as you replace your white spuds with them. You can add different herbs and spices to sweet potatoes, such as cinnamon and rosemary (sweet), or salt, paprika and chilli powder (spicy and savoury), to suit your preference.

A note on rice

While I advocate brown rice over refined white rice, white basmati rice is an exception. It is higher in protein and ▷

---

fibre than regular white rice, and is actually considered a whole grain. This means you can enjoy it guilt-free, as long as you stick to the same portions specified for brown rice in all the meal options in both the Attack and Lifestyle phases. White basmati rice has a lower GI than regular white rice, meaning it is broken down more slowly, keeping your blood-sugar levels stable, in a similar way to brown rice.

High-GI carbs

Foods with a high GI, such as those mentioned under simple carbohydrates (see page 51), are rapidly digested and absorbed by the body, resulting in a spike in blood-sugar levels. When digested, they provide a large amount of glucose, which is usually not used or burnt off soon after, and will most probably be stored as fat, leading to an increase in body fat. By following The Food Effect Diet Vegan you will naturally be avoiding these 'bad' carbs. Better yet, by including the right carbs, the diet will help you to banish cravings for these unhealthy, weight-loss sabotaging carbs, so you'll lose weight and keep it off without even trying.

A high level of insulin, the hormone released in response to glucose in the body, is one of the main contributors to fat storage around the tummy area. Swapping high-GI, refined simple carbohydrates for low-GI, unprocessed complex carbs, helps keep your insulin balanced, making those extra pounds and inches around the waist melt away.

The bottom line: avoiding carbs is not a good idea, no matter what your weight-loss goals are. The most important thing is to review what type of carbs you eat and how much – and The Food Effect Diet Vegan tables and meal plans will guide you on this.

The Food Effect take on sugar

Unless you've been living under a rock, you'll know that sugar is nutrition enemy number one. You'll also know that sugar (or rather the lack of it), plays a key role in losing weight and getting rid of unwanted fat. But is a sugar detox really necessary, and if so, how should you go about it? Here is The Food Effect Diet Vegan way.

Cutting out refined white sugar in its basic, granulated state, as well as in all those highly processed sugary foods and soft drinks (see 'Stay away' in the table relating to carbs on page 32), is certainly essential for losing weight, increasing energy levels, improving skin and mood, getting rid of cellulite, and burning fat. Excluding the things that offer little nutritional value, such as fizzy drinks, is an essential first step in reducing your sugar intake. But is it necessary to cut out fresh fruit (or even dried fruit in specified portion sizes) as we're advised to do by some of the latest fad diets? The answer is no.

You'll see that all fresh fruit (apart from bananas) is included in the 'Eat this' column of the table (see page 26), and even dried fruit is allowed, with portion sizes specified in the meal and snack options. This is because fresh (and dried) fruit provides a wealth of vitamins, minerals and nutrients, and does not have the addictive properties – along with the empty calories – of refined white sugar.

Why avoid bananas?

Although bananas are very nutritious, they are higher in calories and carbohydrate than other fresh fruit; for example, 100g of raw apple contains 52 calories and 14g of carbohydrate, whereas 100g of banana provides 90 calories and 23g of carbohydrate. If you're eating ▶

150–200g of fruit, the calorie and carb count is going to be far higher if you include banana. I don't think it's practical to tell people to have half a banana for a snack – one apple, a pear or orange, for example, is much more practical and realistic. Cutting out bananas and sticking to other fresh fruit has helped so many of my clients reach their weight-loss goals. Many vegan recipes for smoothies or breakfast bowls often include at least one, if not two, bananas, along with other fruit and veg, and possibly nut butter and vegan protein powder. One banana adds an additional 200–250 calories to an already nutrient-dense drink or snack, so you can see why people gain weight from those things without even realising. With so many other nutrient-rich fruit to choose from you won't be missing out.

During the first 28 days (the Attack Phase), the only fruit allowed are apples, oranges, pears, grapefruit and berries. These fruits have the lowest GI, and as this initial phase is designed to wean you off refined sugar and carbohydrates, this will help you to see the effects of reducing your sugar intake. You'll be amazed at the difference it makes to your waistline, mood and energy levels. Occasionally, even during the Attack Phase, a small portion of dried fruit (such as figs or raisins) is specified. Once you move on to the Lifestyle Phase, all types of fruit are allowed, apart from bananas. There are also plenty of delicious, indulgent, yet completely healthy vegan recipes, and suggestions for snacks and sweet treats, once you get on to this phase (see Chapter 12).

The sugary temptations

Fighting off the temptation of delicious-looking vegan desserts, sweets, biscuits, cakes and chocolate bars in virtually every restaurant, supermarket and newsagent (because nowadays vegan products and snacks are widely available) is daunting enough, but even more so when you realise that our brains are actually wired to crave sweet things. This is because refined sugar causes the neurotransmitter dopamine to be released in the brain. Dopamine is associated with our bodies' reward mechanism, so your brain remembers the incentive and signals you to perform the act again (I discuss this in more detail in Chapter 7). Not many people can stop at one biscuit, one sweet or one square of sugar-laden chocolate, but you very rarely hear of people going on an apple binge. Although eating high-GI refined sugary carbs just perpetuates these cravings, fresh fruit does not. It satisfies your sweet tooth in a healthy way, helping to banish cravings and preventing a surge in insulin and dopamine, so conquering cravings and weight gain at the same time.

Sugar has also been found to mimic the effects of opiates in the body. Opiates are addictive chemicals that are used widely for pain management. When a person is addicted to opiates and tries to stop taking them, the body goes into withdrawal. Quitting sugar, especially if you currently consume a lot of it, can cause withdrawal in a similar way. The symptoms can include irritability, fatigue, mood swings, headaches, anger, anxiety and dizziness. Although you're cutting out refined sugary carbs on The Food Effect Diet Vegan, there's no need to cut out healthy fruit and make the process even harder.

The Food Effect Diet Vegan way of eating is specifically designed to make things easy, manageable and enjoyable, unlike extreme sugar-detox diets that make you cut out fruit entirely, leaving you feeling tired, moody, zapped of energy, and too down to find inspiration and motivation to keep going and stick to any plan. With the inclusion of fresh and dried fruit, and low-GI carbs, you might have one or two days of slight difficulty, at worst, when initially cutting out your favourite sweet treats. Over time, however, you'll find that you naturally say no to sugar on a regular basis because you feel better without it. You won't even have to think about avoiding it.

It's important to note that refined sugar can also be hidden in deceptive 'healthy' vegan foods, such as granola, sports drinks and protein bars. Even if you cut out your morning vegan pastry, you might unknowingly fill up on sugar from a seemingly innocent-looking vegan-friendly granola bar or flapjack, which causes the exact same spike in insulin, and the same craving cascade, as junk-filled vegan biscuits, sweets or unhealthy cake. Therefore (fresh fruit aside), it's wise to know where all your sugar intake is coming from. Check the label on packaged cereal, protein bars and snacks, and if sugar is listed in the first three ingredients (note: this includes sugar in its various forms such as sucrose, glucose syrup, high fructose corn syrup, etc.), avoid the product altogether. And remember that vegan does not necessarily mean healthy: I've seen 'vegan, gluten-free, dairy-free' cookies that are packed with sugar, margarine, trans fats and palm oil. Be label savvy, and don't be fooled by clever marketing and food companies trying to trick consumers by writing 'vegan' across the package.

Juices – not so healthy

Fruit smoothies and juices are another thing to be wary of. These cause a completely different reaction in the body compared to eating fresh fruit. They can easily contain more sugar than you should consume at once, so if you drink too many of them you might be fighting off sugar cravings for an entire day. Fruit juice is basically sugared water, with all the fibre from the fruit extracted and very little vitamin and mineral content remaining. This is why fruit juice is not included in The Food Effect Diet Vegan plan, and is under the 'Stay away' column in the tables.

Now you know what you're up against, what can you do about it? Fortunately, it's very easy to break the sugar-craving cycle on

The Food Effect Diet Vegan plan. Simply avoid all the foods in the 'Stay away' column of the tables, and follow the suggested meal and snack options instead. You'll be off the sweet stuff and on to a better, healthier, slimmer you in no time.

Sweeteners – take the scare stories with a pinch of salt

Although the inclusion of fruit and whole-grain carbs will help to keep you satisfied during your weight-loss journey, some of us have a naturally sweet tooth that needs to be satisfied, and although you definitely won't be allowed to sprinkle sugar on your cereal, why should you have to go without enjoying the taste when there's a perfectly safe and calorie-free way to do so? Additionally, having a large mug of sweet coffee or herbal tea can go a long way in helping to beat sugar cravings.

Although xylitol and stevia might sound like sci-fi villains that people automatically assume are unhealthy, they are actually perfectly safe, natural sugar substitutes, or sweeteners. Fears about their potentially toxic effects, ranging from diabetes, cancer, strokes and seizures to vomiting, high blood pressure and dizziness, have all been cited, but none of these claims have actually been proven. The American Food and Drug Administration and the European Food Safety Authority, who investigate these substances in depth, say they're completely safe, and I'd similarly advise you to take the scare stories with a pinch of salt. Real sugar is far worse for your weight and health in so many respects, and that's definitely been proven.

Stevia (my preference) is completely natural, as it is derived from a plant, and tastes far sweeter than processed sugar, so the amount needed to create the same level of sweetness is dramatically lower. Even better, it contains virtually zero calories and no nasties, and doesn't spike blood-sugar levels at all – making it the best option all round.

So many of my clients are scared of sweeteners, such as stevia, yet they spoon regular refined white sugar into their tea or coffee and feed it to their children. This makes absolutely no sense – refined white sugar (sucrose), with its high calorie content and need for insulin to break it down, poses the real risk of weight gain, obesity and type-2 diabetes. Sweeteners, on the other hand, have zero (or very few) calories, do not raise insulin levels and are approved as safe for diabetics. As these sweeteners are absorbed more slowly than sugar, they do not contribute to high blood-sugar levels or the resulting hyperglycaemia caused by an insufficient insulin response. This characteristic has also proven beneficial for people suffering from metabolic syndrome (a common disorder in our Western society), which includes insulin resistance (that can lead to type-2 diabetes), hypertension, hypercholesterolemia and an increased risk of blood clots.

Interestingly, the sweetener xylitol is actively beneficial for dental health. It not only reduces cavities but numerous studies have shown that xylitol is effective in inducing remineralisation of deep layers of demineralised enamel in the teeth. This is because the perception of sweetness from consuming xylitol causes the secretion of saliva, which acts as a buffer against the acidic environment created by the micro-organisms in dental plaque. The increase in salivation can return an acidic pH to a neutral range within a few minutes of xylitol consumption.

Interestingly, sufficient evidence has also found that xylitol (in chewing gum, lozenges, nasal spray, and so on) reduces the incidence of acute middle-ear infection in healthy children.

Artificial sweeteners

Although both the American Food and Drug Administration and the European Food Safety Authority approve the use of artificial sweeteners including aspartame (Equal) and saccharin (Sweet 'n Low), these are completely unnatural and made purely from artificial chemicals. I would avoid these and advise sticking to only the natural sugar substitutes (that is, stevia and xylitol).

You'll see that the addition of sweeteners such as stevia or xylitol (as well as all-natural ground cinnamon) is suggested in the meal options. You can rest assured that you'll be doing your health and weight a favour by cutting out refined white sugar and using these natural sweeteners instead.

Syrups

Agave nectar syrup and pure maple syrup are also natural sweeteners that will tingle your taste buds. Coconut nectar honey is another delicious and healthy vegan alternative to real honey. These are included and allowed in moderation in The Food Effect Diet Vegan plan. They're rich in calcium, iron, B vitamins and potassium, and are certainly better for you than the processed sugar found in sweets and unhealthy baked goods. As they're higher in calories, however, their amounts are limited and specified (unlike for calorie-free stevia) in the meal options.

In short, if you have a sweet tooth and like your coffee, tea, porridge and dairy-free natural yoghurts to taste sweet, go ahead and add some natural Food Effect-friendly sweetener. A bit of stevia is far better than sugar.

Wheat and gluten – a few more myths debunked

'Wheat makes you fat' and 'removing gluten from your diet will help you lose weight' are two popular nutrition myths that you may have heard, but there is absolutely no medical or scientific basis for this to be the case for the average healthy individual.

The world of health and fitness is awash with misinformation. I see so many clients who have been exposed to repeated misinformation, and have gone 'gluten-free' for no real reason, with the result that they are then left with very restrictive diets and even a fear of certain foods. (I am not, however, referring to those who have a genuine intolerance to wheat or gluten, and might need to eliminate them accordingly.)

The myth that 'wheat makes you fat' is in part a result of the so-called 'clean-eating' diet craze, which blames wheat for obesity and a host of other medical conditions, with people making unsubstantiated claims that cutting out gluten cured all their ailments. Yes, people who eat a lot of refined wheat flour in foods such as white bread, biscuits and pastries will indeed gain weight; and yes, if they cut out these refined foods and eat a more balanced diet (as you will be doing on The Food Effect Diet Vegan) they'll lose weight and feel better. But it's not because of the wheat; it's because they've improved their overall diet and meal balance, and cut out refined carbs and sugar. There have been no scientific studies that support wheat as the culprit for our obesity epidemic or that support a wheat-free diet for weight loss. The best thing you can do for weight loss is to replace refined white wheat (such as that in white bread, vegan pastries, cakes, biscuits and muffins made with refined white flour) with whole grains (like wholemeal bread, or vegan muffins made with wholemeal flour or other unrefined flours), to increase your fibre intake so that you'll feel fuller and avoid cravings.

In terms of gluten, increasing diagnoses of coeliac disease (a true gluten intolerance), due to heightened awareness and better screening, has put gluten in the spotlight in recent years; however, many people mistakenly think that a gluten-free diet is the key to weight loss. This couldn't be further from the truth. People are blaming gluten for symptoms when it's not the underlying cause. It's trendy, and many celebrities have endorsed gluten-free diets, so people jump on the bandwagon. Going on a gluten-free diet can be unnecessarily expensive, and will not guarantee better health or weight loss. There is no evidence to suggest that weight or fitness is improved in any way when following a gluten-free diet.

In fact, a recent study in the *Journal of the American Medical Association* (*JAMA*), as well as other studies, showed that the growing popularity of gluten-free diets, endorsed by high-profile celebrities, has been driven by fashion choices rather than diagnosed health problems. Researchers found that there has been no increase in the numbers of those suffering from coeliac disease in the past six years, yet those on gluten-free diets have risen threefold. The authors say that other reasons are also clearly driving the trend, including a misinformed public perception that gluten-free diets are healthier, and people are increasingly self-diagnosing themselves with gluten sensitivity without having the typical symptoms of coeliac disease. The studies confirm that, unsurprisingly, the rising popularity of gluten-free diets is not accounted for by any increase in clinically proven cases of coeliac disease. The huge number of gluten-free foods now available on supermarket shelves is also helping to boost the numbers of those shunning wheat. Although only 1 per cent of the UK population is estimated to be affected by coeliac disease, 55 per cent of the market is made up of non-sufferers. More than half the UK population is now buying gluten-free products, so savvy marketing also plays a huge role in influencing food choices.

Gluten-free diets are specifically designed for the 1 per cent of the population that does have coeliac disease and the 6 per cent with non-coeliac gluten sensitivity. For these people, foods containing gluten, such as wheat, rye and barley, can lead to a host of symptoms including gastrointestinal problems, skin rashes and anaemia. For the rest of the population, however, gluten should not pose a problem. Whole-grain wheat, barley and rye are nutritional powerhouses; they are good sources of fibre, B vitamins, vitamin E, iron, magnesium and antioxidants – all of which are essential for healthy living and disease prevention, especially for vegans who already have a more restrictive diet, albeit for good reasons.

Additionally, many gluten-free products are higher in calories and other unhealthy ingredients than their gluten-containing counterparts (as well as being much more expensive), but people are conned into thinking that anything with a 'gluten-free' label must be healthier and will help with weight loss, when this is nothing more than a myth.

The Food Effect Diet Vegan is the last diet that you will ever need. As you can see, you will no longer be focusing on avoiding carbohydrates or gluten, as so many other diets will have you do. On The Food Effect Diet Vegan, you'll be eating plenty of carbohydrates in order to start dropping pounds.

CHAPTER 4

The Food Effect Diet Vegan Guide to Protein

More than just beans and tofu

Vegan proteins are more varied than people often think, but before we get on to some of the best protein sources, below are some basic facts on the science of protein.

What is protein?

If you were to ask most people what protein is, how the body uses it and what foods are good sources of it, most would answer that it's used to build muscle and is found in meat, chicken and eggs. Now although none of that is inaccurate, it's just the tip of the iceberg when it comes to protein. Proteins aren't solely required to help the body build muscle, and they certainly aren't only found in meat and eggs – thankfully. They are required for virtually every bodily function. They are the primary building blocks of the body. Our muscles are made from protein, but so are our skin, hair, nails, eyes, bones and all our organs. Additionally, our hormones, enzymes and blood cells are mainly made up of proteins. Together with water, protein is the most abundant substance in the human body. Although, of course, I won't be advocating any animal protein in this book, I certainly think that protein is essential and you definitely won't be skimping on it, even on a vegan diet. I've put countless hours and brainpower into ensuring that no meals or any day on The Food Effect Diet Vegan will be lacking in protein.

How much protein do you need?

As mentioned above, protein is essential for virtually every bodily function. That being said, I think our society has also become a bit protein crazy, and there are new products being fortified with protein everyday, when really most of us probably consume enough protein without even trying. Being vegan does mean needing to pay more attention to ensuring you're consuming enough protein. Although fortified products, such as a vegan protein powder, might be extremely helpful, especially if you work out a lot or train intensely, I certainly don't believe that we need to be buying protein-fortified loaves of bread, breakfast cereal or protein water (yes, it exists). You can get all the protein you need on a healthy whole-food, plant-based diet and, as mentioned earlier, your protein needs have already been worked out for you in The Food Effect Diet Vegan plan and meal options.

Although you don't need to do any calculations, or track or measure anything, the way to calculate how much protein you need, even just for interest, is by using the RNI (reference nutrient intake) calculation. This is 0.75 × your body weight in kilograms. It's important to note that this is the *minimum* you need to be consuming each day. It is safe to go up to double the RNI for protein. And in certain stages of life, such as during pregnancy and while breastfeeding, or if someone is more active, it might be beneficial to consume closer to the higher number. For a 55kg woman, for example, that will be 0.75 × 55 = 41g

of protein a day: not very much. And a 70kg male would be
0.75 × 70 = 52g of protein. That's basically 2½ vegetable burgers. (Note that the calculation is for the *protein element* of the
food and not the weight of the food itself.) And remember that
whole grains, nuts, chia seeds, spinach, soya milk and yoghurts,
pulses and virtually everything you consume contains protein, so
it's actually very easy for vegans to meet their protein needs on
a healthy diet. Although you won't have to do any of the maths,
as all your meal options are very clearly laid out in the 28-day
Food Effect Attack Phase and in the Lifestyle Phase, here is some
information that illustrates how it's possible to meet your protein
requirements without consuming meat.

Vegan-friendly foods high in protein

Food	Protein amount
25g (1 scoop) vegan protein powder	20–30g protein
75g cooked lentils	18g protein
75g cooked split peas	16g protein
40g chia seeds	12g protein
100g cooked edamame beans	11g protein
200g soya yoghurt	10g protein
120g (½ tin) cooked chickpeas	9g protein
30g peanuts	8g protein
30g (2 tbsp) pumpkin seeds	8g protein
1 cup/250ml unsweetened soya milk	8g protein
30g (2 tbsp) sunflower seeds	7g protein
100g cooked peas	7g protein
100g uncooked oats	7g protein
130g cooked kidney beans (tinned)	6g protein
125g cooked quinoa	6g protein
30g cashew nuts	6g protein
125g cooked spinach	4.3g protein
1 sweet potato	4g protein

In essence, it's virtually impossible to become protein deficient on a well-balanced, plant-based diet.

Eating plenty of protein throughout the day (along with whole grains, fruit, vegetables and healthy fats), as laid out later in this book, will improve your body composition, promote satiety, increase calorie burning and improve insulin control. All your meal and snack options in both phases of The Food Effect Diet Vegan have been perfectly designed to do this.

Vegan milks and cheeses

Let's look at a few protein-containing foods that have been the subject of controversy and confusion.

Dairy alternatives and plant-based milks

I need to start off by saying that I am in no way anti-dairy, and I myself (being pescatarian) do consume dairy foods such as Greek yoghurt and cottage cheese. Of course, this book is written specifically for vegans or those wishing to adopt a vegan or more plant-based lifestyle, and while I do believe that there's no harm in consuming dairy, I just as much believe that one can meet all the same nutritional needs without it. It simply requires a bit more thought and knowledge, all of which will be explained here.

Dairy milk contains calcium, which is an essential nutrient for our bodies, not just for bone and teeth health, but to maintain a healthy weight, too. Cutting back on the amount of calcium-containing foods you eat can actually signal the body to make more fat cells. When you don't have enough calcium, your body tries to hold on to whatever's there. This triggers the release of a compound called calcitriol, which, according to a study in the *American Journal of Clinical Nutrition*, increases the production of fat cells.

Although this might sound worrying to you as a vegan, rest assured that there are plenty of non-dairy foods that are rich sources of calcium, as well as many great calcium-fortified milks and products on the market. Non-dairy foods such as almonds, sesame seeds, tahini and spinach are amazing sources of calcium. For vegans, these should be a key part of your daily diet. My advice is to aim for three portions of calcium-containing foods each day. This can include calcium-fortified plant-based milk or yoghurt with breakfast, a handful of almonds and fruit as a snack, a serving of tofu or edamame beans in a salad at lunch, and dark green leafy vegetables, such as spinach and broccoli, with supper in the evening. That's all very manageable.

Thankfully, you don't need to even think about this, as these foods have already been included in The Food Effect Diet Vegan meal options, ensuring all your calcium needs are met.

Recommended daily intakes of calcium are slightly higher for adolescents than for any other age group due to their rapid bone growth, and because these are the years when bone structure is laid down for life. But this remains an important nutrient for everyone, right up to old age. Men and women over the age of 19 need 700–1,000mg of calcium per day. A cup of fortified almond milk, for example, provides 240mg, and foods like tahini and tofu are even richer sources of calcium than actual milk.

Although after the age of 21 we no longer build bone density, we can help to maintain it by keeping up our calcium intake. Consuming sufficient calcium-rich foods can help to protect against osteoporosis in later life. Calcium also helps maintain muscle mass, which improves metabolism, helping you to burn calories more efficiently throughout the day.

Aside from the importance of protein and calcium for bone health, vitamin D is another essential nutrient that is strongly linked to calcium. It is commonly known as the 'sunshine vitamin', but sadly those of us living in the UK – or in any country that's not hot and sunny all year round – can't rely on sunshine to provide this essential nutrient. Low levels of vitamin D have been associated with increased fat storage, among many other health problems (see also page 154). Vitamin D deficiency also causes the brain to issue hunger-signalling hormones, tempting you to reach for the biscuit tin and sugary sweets. Additionally, calcium-rich diets have been found to aid weight loss, but vitamin D is required to regulate calcium absorption. Thankfully, most plant-based milks are fortified with calcium *and* vitamin D, making them a real win-win. Make sure to check the labels of any dairy-free milks and yoghurts you buy, to ensure they're fortified with calcium and vitamin D.

Additionally, aim for a plant-based milk with no added sugar. There are many great options on the market.

For all these reasons you'll see plenty of dairy alternative options (such as almond milk and dairy-free soya yoghurts) in The Food Effect Diet Vegan Attack Phase and Lifestyle Phase meal options. Highly processed coconut or soya oil-based 'cheeses' are not allowed due to their high saturated fat and calorie content.

A note on non-dairy (vegan) cheeses

There is now an incredible amount of vegan cheeses available on the market. Although this is great, it's important to note that there is a *lot* of bad along with the good. Many vegan cream cheeses and hard cheeses made from coconut oil are extremely high in fat and calories, along with artificial flavourings, preservatives and thickeners added.

While coconut oil is healthy in moderation and great to cook with, I'd avoid vegan cheeses made predominantly from it, as the calories and saturated fat content adds up and it also provides very little in the way of protein or calcium – not a great substitute for the few health benefits (protein and calcium) of eating real cheese.

Almond- and cashew-based non-dairy cheeses (for example, Nush Almond Milk cheeses and Kite Hill from the US) are, however, great vegan alternatives. They provide decent levels of protein and are low in calories and saturated fat.

Which plant-based milk to choose?

Of all the dairy-free milks now available, from hemp to hazelnut, and oat to almond milk, deciding which plant-based milk to choose can be rather challenging. Gone are the days when they were a reluctant replacement for cow's milk. Now more and more people (non-vegans included) are choosing plant-based milks for their unique tastes, and the health benefits they provide.

Dairy-free milks are generally very low in saturated fat (unlike full-fat dairy) that can contribute to raised blood cholesterol levels, not to mention calories and weight gain, when consumed in excess. What's more, many have specific health benefits (for example, nut milks are rich in vitamin E) and are fortified with calcium and vitamin D, the bone building nutrients, along with vitamin B12, which can be hard to get enough of (without supplementation) on a vegan diet.

It is important to note, however, that some are not fortified with calcium, and many are highly sweetened with added sugar, so make sure to choose one that is fortified and has no added sugar (there are plenty on the market).

Here's a quick summary of some of the most popular types of dairy-free milks.

Soya milk Scientists at McGill University in Quebec found that soya milks trumped other dairy-free alternatives nutritionally. Soya milk has as much protein as cow's milk, and is low in calories, and many are fortified with vitamins and minerals, too, making it a great choice as a dairy alternative. Many tend to be sweetened with sugar, however, so look for 'unsweetened' on the label. If you are concerned about consuming soya, read 'Soya – debunking the myths' a bit further on in this chapter.

Almond milk Commercially, almond milk is made by blending 2 per cent almonds with water. Many people make their own at home by soaking almonds, blending them with water and then straining the liquid. Although this works well, it doesn't work out to be cheaper (almonds are expensive, and you only end up keeping the water from them) and it won't be fortified with all the essential vitamins and minerals that many on the market contain. I'd advise buying an unsweetened almond milk instead. It's rich in vitamin E and antioxidants, important for protecting the body's cells against damage (which lead to ageing, heart disease and cancers). The one downside is that it's low in protein, with a 200ml glass providing just 1 gram of protein; however, if your diet is rich in protein from other sources (as it will be if you follow The Food Effect Diet Vegan meal plan and options), you needn't be concerned about this, as you'll be consuming sufficient protein to meet your needs every day. Almond milk is very mild tasting, making it perfect to use in tea and coffee, as well as in cereals and porridge. As it's so widely available, with fortified unsweetened options on the market, and very low in calories (just 13 calories per 100ml) it's the non-dairy milk that I've specified in most of the meal options and recipes.

Hemp milk is made from a blend of hemp seeds, water and a touch of sea salt. It's rich in essential omega-3 fatty acids (one cup of hemp milk contains more omega-3s than a tuna steak) making it fantastic for vegans. In my opinion, it looks and tastes the most similar to cow's milk – and also has a slightly sweet taste despite containing no added sugar or artificial sweeteners. It's low in calories, too (26 calories per 100ml). If you come across it, it's definitely allowed on The Food Effect Diet Vegan. I haven't included it in meal plans simply because it can be difficult to find.

Oat milk is made by soaking and blending steel-cut or rolled oats (or gluten-free oats to make gluten-free oat milk) with water and then straining them through muslin to separate the milk from the oats. It's a good source of beta-glucan oat fibre, which studies have shown can help to lower cholesterol; however, it's not as nutritious as eating whole oats. It's become hugely popular in coffee chains as an alternative to dairy milk. Oat milk generally has more calories and carbs than almond, soya or hemp milk while providing less protein than soya and dairy milk. Although the most popular commercial brands are fortified with calcium, vitamin D and the B vitamins, it usually has added rapeseed or vegetable oil, and comes in at 46 calories per 100ml. It's fine to have occasionally, but it wouldn't be the milk I'd advise for daily consumption.

Rice milk Made in a similar way to oat milk, but using brown rice instead of oats, this has natural enzymes added to break down the starch into sugars, giving it a subtly sweet taste. Most brands contain some added sunflower or vegetable oil, so it has the same calories as semi-skimmed milk, but without the protein.

Coconut milk in a carton (used as a dairy-free alternative to milk) is a less creamy, lower fat version of canned coconut milk. It's made by blending the white coconut flesh with water or coconut water. Coconut milk contains some medium chain saturated fats, which, unlike regular saturated fat, have been credited with improved fat loss when consumed as part of a weight-loss plan, as well as having many other health benefits, such as improving the gut microbiome. It's delicious in smoothies, healthy vegan desserts and breakfast recipes such as pancakes and chia seed pudding. It's definitely fine and healthy to use for these, or when specified in a recipe.

Soya – debunking the myths

Most of you will have heard the ongoing nutritional controversy and dietary myths surrounding soya, earning it a bad reputation in recent years, largely for no good reason. Healthy, non-GMO (genetically modified) soya and soya-based products in fact provide numerous health benefits, especially in a vegan diet.

Soya is a fantastic source of important nutrients including protein, calcium and B vitamins, and the downside of not getting enough protein and calcium in your diet (which can easily happen by cutting out all healthy soya-based foods on a vegan diet) can be harmful to everything from weight, blood-sugar levels, muscles, bone density and more. On top of this, there is endless research showing that soya in your diet can help to lower cholesterol and reduce the risk of heart disease and various cancers.

Several epidemiological studies have found that soya protein might reduce the risk for cancers including breast, colon and prostate. Studies show that women who include soya products in their diet are less likely to develop breast cancer, compared with women who don't.

A study published in *JAMA* reported results based on 5,042 women previously diagnosed with breast cancer who were participating in the Shanghai Breast Cancer Survival Study. The study showed that women who regularly consumed soya products, such as soya milk, tofu or edamame, had a 32 per cent lower risk of recurrence and a 29 per cent decreased risk of death, compared with women who consumed little or no soya. Meanwhile, a study at Kaiser Permanente healthcare centre in America suggested much the same thing. Women who avoid soya products receive no advantage at all, whereas those who include soya products in their diets appear to cut their risk of cancer recurrence.

Despite all this evidence, its consumption is still not without controversy and a large amount of scaremongering. The cause of the controversy surrounding soya is mainly due to its phytoestrogen content.

The phytoestrogen factor

Phytoestrogens (plant oestrogens) are plant-derived compounds found in a wide variety of foods, most notably soya. Many health benefits, including a decreased risk of osteoporosis, heart disease, breast cancer and menopausal symptoms, are frequently attributed to phytoestrogens, but many are also considered endocrine disruptors due to their actions on oestrogen receptors in the body.

Because the structure of isoflavones (the phytoestrogens found in soya) is similar to oestrogen, high levels of which are associated with breast cancer, many fear that the body might mistake isoflavones as oestrogen, thus increasing the risk of breast cancer. But our body is not that simple. Women actually have two oestrogen receptors: alpha and beta. The alpha receptor causes cells to grow, which means that if an isoflavone binds to the alpha receptor it could increase a woman's risk of developing breast cancer. But binding to beta receptors creates the opposite effect, and isoflavones preferentially bind to the beta receptors, which might explain why consuming soya has been linked to lower rates of breast cancer.

One recent study found that women who ate the most soya isoflavones had a 24 per cent lower risk of developing breast cancer than those who didn't eat soya.

Although isoflavones are similar in structure to oestrogen, they contain anti-oestrogen properties, which means that they can block natural oestrogens in the body from binding to an oestrogen receptor (like those found in the breasts or uterus), thus protecting women from the effects of excess levels of oestrogen. In addition to this, they have both antioxidant and anti-inflammatory properties and can work in other ways to reduce cancer growth. A study from Tufts University found that not only is soya safe, but it might also inhibit the development and recurrence of breast cancer cells.

A famous American media doctor, Dr Eric Berg, explains

phytoestrogens and answers the question of whether consuming foods that contain phytoestrogens will increase your oestrogen levels. The answer is no, not more than you already have in your body. Phytoestrogens only block receptors for bad oestrogen, which automatically raises your relative good oestrogen circulating in the body. *But* it will not increase your overall levels higher than you already have.

Soya and men

As for men who are concerned, soya products have been shown to have no adverse effects on men and may even help to prevent cancer in them. A meta-analysis published in *Fertility and Sterility*, based on more than 50 treatment groups, showed that neither soya products nor isoflavone supplements from soya affect testosterone levels in men, whereas another study showed that increased intake of soya resulted in a 26 per cent reduction in prostate cancer risk.

Cancer-fighting foods

Consuming soya milk, soya yoghurts, tofu or edamame beans, for example, is safe for both men and women.

The American Institute for Cancer Research recommends soya as a cancer-fighting food, as it is associated with a decreased risk of breast cancer recurrence and mortality. Studies have also found that consuming soya early in life, during childhood or adolescence, might lower the lifetime risk of developing breast cancer, and that populations consuming the most soya have the lowest rates of breast cancer.

Soya and weight

Moving away from the more serious myths surrounding soya, some people have also been concerned about weight gain. But studies actually suggest that soya milk consumed in moderation can help you to lose weight by mimicking the hormones in the body that reduce hunger, namely leptin, a hormone that signals to the brain that you are full.

A study from the University of Illinois found that when rats were injected with soya protein, they lost weight despite having unlimited access to food. Another study presented at the Annual Meeting of the Society for the Study of Ingestive Behavior, concluded that soya prevents postmenopausal weight gain in female rats, likely due to its oestrogen-like compounds.

In short, soya is most definitely safe in moderation and contributes various health benefits and nutrients, such as calcium and protein, which are both important to incorporate in a vegan diet.

The Food Effect Diet Vegan meal plan and options are very low in soya (and definitely contain no unhealthy GMO soya) due to its variety of whole plant-based foods. There is certainly no excess soya for you to worry about. And a bit of healthy soya yoghurt and some tofu-based recipes will be far more beneficial to your overall weight, health and nutritional needs than unnecessarily cutting them all out.

Vegan protein favourites

Here are some other great, nutritious vegan sources of protein, the benefits of which are outlined below.

Chickpeas

These pulses are a fantastic source of fibre and protein, and have a low glycaemic index (see page 52). This powerful combination makes them particularly good at helping with weight management. In an Australian study, adults who ate 100g of chickpeas a day for four weeks ate fewer processed snack foods and felt fuller, compared to when they didn't include chickpeas in their daily diets. One 165g serving of cooked chickpeas provides 50 per cent of your daily fibre requirement, so it's no wonder that this legume provides long-lasting energy, keeps you feeling full, promotes good digestion, curbs appetite and has even been shown to help lower LDL (bad) cholesterol. There are plenty of delicious meal options and recipes incorporating chickpeas in Chapters 11, 12 and 13.

Lentils

These little legumes are heavenly, healthy, hearty and filling. Just 100g (raw weight) of lentils packs in 80 per cent of your daily requirement of fibre, which increases satiety and steadies blood-sugar levels. Lentils are not only packed with protein, but they are also an excellent source of folate, which has been shown to be a key nutrient in preventing and treating depression, insomnia and muscular fatigue. Lentils are available in a variety of colours, and all pack a nutritional punch. Add them to salads, stews or pasta dishes, and try my recipe for Easiest-Ever Red Lentil Soup (see page 258).

Quinoa

One of the few vegan foods that is a complete protein, quinoa contains all nine essential amino acids. It's also a rich source of fibre, magnesium, folate, copper, thiamin and vitamin B6. It is included in plenty of the meal options in both the Attack and Lifestyle Phases, and there are many delicious quinoa-based recipes in Chapter 13.

Tofu

Made from soya bean curd, tofu provides a complete source of vegan protein as well as many essential minerals, including calcium. There are two types of tofu: Japanese-style silken tofu, which is undrained and unprocessed and has a smoother, more custard-like texture. This can be used in desserts, dressings and dips. The other more commonly used type is Chinese-style tofu, where the curds are pressed into blocks. This can range in texture from soft to extra firm. Look out for firm or extra firm to add to soups, or bake, grill, pan-fry (with minimal oil) or add to stir-fries. It's best to buy a non-flavoured version and season it yourself so that you know exactly what goes into it (there are some delicious recipes using tofu in Chapter 13). Add it to a vegetable stir-fry or salads for a nutritious plant-based vegan meal.

Peanut butter

One serving of this tasty spread contains 5g of healthy monounsaturated fatty acids, which research shows can help to keep you slimmer and keep belly fat at bay (see more on fats and the health benefits of nuts in Chapter 6). Almond and cashew butters are equally healthy, delicious alternatives. A 2 tbsp serving of nut butter contains about 7g of protein, not to mention a host of vitamins, minerals and heart-healthy fats. Spread your choice of nut butter on to cut-up fresh fruit (such as apple slices) or vegetables, or whole-grain crackers, and you've got yourself a delicious, satisfying snack in minutes.

Cashew nuts

These are my all-time favourite nuts. As well as being a great source of protein, cashew nuts contain a host of essential vitamins and minerals, including magnesium, copper, manganese, phosphorus and vitamin K. This combination makes them ideal for promoting bone and muscle strength, preventing migraines, improving memory, lowering blood pressure and reducing the risk of heart disease and cancer. They're so incredibly versatile – you can snack on a handful of raw cashews (you'll see this one included often in The Food Effect meal plan) and they're great in vegan recipes, such as raw balls and desserts (see Chapter 13), or to make a savoury sauce.

Pumpkin seeds

Next time you're craving something crunchy, instead of opening a bag of unhealthy crisps, grab some dry-roasted pumpkin seeds instead. A generous 28g serving packs in 8g of belly-filling protein, plus each little seed is a great source of fibre, vitamins, minerals, heart-healthy fats and antioxidants.

Chia Seeds

Chia seeds are an amazing source of omega-3 fatty acids and are also packed with protein, fibre, iron and calcium. This combination makes them good for blood-sugar control and weight loss. A study by Canadian scientists found that chia seeds helped patients with type-2 diabetes lose weight. It's thought that chia seeds aid weight loss by increasing levels of adiponectin, a protein involved in the breakdown of fat. They are incredibly versatile: they can be soaked to make a delicious breakfast pudding, added to raw balls and muesli mixes, or sprinkled onto vegan yoghurt or salads. They're now widely available in most major supermarkets. Try my recipes for Chocolate Chia Seed Pudding and Blueberry Chia Seed Jam (see Chapter 13) – both make a delicious, healthy and satisfying breakfast or sweet treat.

Nutritional yeast

Not only is this absolutely jam-packed with nutritional goodness (as its name suggests), but it's also totally delicious. Although I am not vegan, I choose this over dairy cheese to add to soups, sauces, pastas and more, all the time. It's packed with protein, B vitamins, fibre and iron. It's low in fat and calories, and free of salt, sugar and gluten. Making it suitable for all. Although it's naturally rich in B vitamins, it's now available fortified with vitamin B12 and vitamin D, making it even more of a nutritional winner. It's available in most health-food shops.

Spinach

Yes, spinach. It isn't a mistake including this one in The Food Effect Diet Vegan top protein choices. Protein accounts for 30 per cent of the calories in spinach, and it contains a significant 3g of protein per 100g (uncooked weight). It's also packed with other essential nutrients including iron, folate, magnesium, vitamins A, B2, B6, C, E, K and calcium, manganese, potassium and zinc. It also contains dietary fibre, copper and phosphorus. These are more than enough good reasons to be eating your spinach. It's included in many of the meal options and recipes in this book, so your protein will not only be coming from the more traditional vegan sources such as chickpeas, beans, tofu and lentils, but even your salad leaves will provide a substantial dose of protein.

Jackfruit

A large green fruit from South-east Asia, jackfruit has recently become popular as a substitute for meat. It's highly nutritious, packed with fibre, iron, calcium, B vitamins, particularly vitamin B6, potassium and magnesium. You can buy it canned in water or brine. It's super-reasonably priced (at just over £1 for a tin) and is available in most big supermarkets. Jackfruit is low in sugar, virtually fat-free and a good source of protein. It is also rich in carotenoids, vitamin C and flavones, which are all anti-inflammatory and reduce the risk of chronic disease such as heart disease and cancer. The fibre in jackfruit helps to improve digestion and prevent constipation, and because it's high in Food Effect-friendly complex carbs, it provides a boost of energy

without disrupting your blood-sugar levels. Clinical trials conducted at Sydney University's Glycemic Index Research Service
(SUGiRS) found that raw jackfruit has a lower glycaemic load
than both wheat or rice. Jackfruit doesn't have a strong flavour
or taste on its own, so it is able to soak up herbs, spices and other
flavourings. This allows the fruit to be made into plant-based
versions of shredded chicken, pulled pork or other meat-based
meals, as well as a variety of sweet and savoury dishes. Try my
recipe for Pulled Barbecue Jackfruit and Barbecue Jackfruit
Burgers (Chapter 13).

As you can see, The Food Effect Diet Vegan encourages you to
eat from a wide variety of plant-based proteins while reducing
protein alternatives that are high in saturated fat, such as highly
processed vegan cheeses made predominantly from coconut oil.
Many people think that vegan protein means just beans or tofu,
but hopefully this chapter has shown you that you can meet your
protein requirements from a wide range of sources, as well as
your calcium and vitamin D intake with dairy-free alternatives.

With this diet, you'll be relying on the healthiest protein
choices, thereby promoting weight loss and keeping you full,
slim and satisfied.

CHAPTER 5

Not Eating Red Meat

The key to health, longevity and weight loss ... even for non-vegans

As you're reading this book, you probably don't need convincing to avoid red meat; however, there may be some readers who are just dipping their toes into veganism and wish to explore a more plant-based lifestyle without going totally vegan. This chapter might provide some inspiration if you're looking for an added incentive to adopt a more plant-based lifestyle. Or, as a vegan, you might be interested to know why I advocate cutting out red meat even for my non-vegan clients. My first book, *The Food Effect Diet*, doesn't advocate cutting out anything else, so why red meat?

If you're new to veganism, or still following a flexitarian approach and just trying to reduce your red meat intake, you'll be assured to know that I've seen countless meat-loving clients, who have looked at me as if they thought I was either crazy or joking when I told them that they would be cutting out red meat once they start their Food Effect plan. They told me that there was no way they could do it. I made sure that I gave them plenty of alternatives, just as I have here, in The Food Effect Diet Vegan meal plans and recipes. And guess what? After a few weeks they came back having lost weight, telling me that they'd never felt better, and that they weren't even tempted by the red meat options in restaurants or at dinners served at friends' homes.

Although I advise cutting out red meat and adopting a more plant-based lifestyle, if you aren't vegan already, this doesn't have to mean that it's something you should never have again, if that's not what you want. I'm all about balance, and I believe that each person should do what works best for themself. Even reducing your red meat intake and adopting a more flexitarian approach will bring tremendous health, weight loss (and environmental) benefits. What you gain is so much more than what you give up. Of course, if you're vegan and don't eat red meat already, hopefully you'll find the following to be interesting reading about the health benefits of your chosen lifestyle, and perhaps you can share some insights with non-vegan friends and family members.

More than just meat-free Monday

Many people have been making the argument that our population has grown fat because we eat too much starch and sugar, and not enough meat, butter and fat. Recently the news has been full of articles citing research that saturated fat does not cause heart disease, as was once believed. The predictable headlines followed: 'Eat Bacon and Butter'.

Alas, I have to tell you that bacon and red meat, especially processed meats, are anything but health foods. They might not be proven to directly cause heart disease but there is certainly enough conclusive evidence that they cause many other diseases, and they do nothing to help with weight loss. Moreover, obesity certainly does cause an endless list of health risks, including heart disease, diabetes, stroke, cancer and more. As mentioned earlier, I've seen the positive effects that cutting out red meat has had on hundreds of clients, and now I'd like to share that information with you, too. Not only does eating red meat make you gain weight, it also affects your overall appearance.

Eating large quantities of red meat on a regular basis can seriously affect your skin and body's ageing process, as it has been shown to be particularly inflammatory for the skin. By cutting out red meat you'll be doing your health and weight a great favour.

Nearly a third of people reduced their meat consumption during 2016, according to figures from the British Social Attitudes survey, as they tried to heed health warnings about processed foods such as bacon, ham and sausages. Forty-four per cent have cut back, plan to do so or are vegetarian already. Experts say that consumption is likely to fall further after the World Health Organization (WHO) classified bacon, sausages and processed meats as 'group 1 carcinogens' – in the same category as alcohol and cigarettes – and ranked red meat, including beef and pork, as the next level down: 'probably carcinogenic'. The NHS says that too much red meat and processed meat can increase the likelihood of bowel cancer, with just two rashers a day raising the risk by a whopping 18 per cent.

Along with this very valid reason for cutting down on meat consumption for health reasons, as well as the benefits of it being more economical, The Food Effect lifestyle advises cutting out red meat for weight loss, too.

When I first founded my nutrition practice and started seeing clients, my advice to cut out red meat was primarily driven by concerns about health and what I viewed as clear evidence that doing so was beneficial for health (blood pressure, cholesterol, cancer and heart-disease risk), despite what others out there were promoting. I placed all red meat in the 'Stay away' column in The Food Effect tables, and advised all my non-vegan clients to replace red meat with poultry, eggs, fish and low-fat dairy foods, as well as pulses and other plant-based sources of protein. As a result, clients returned with improved blood results, lowered cholesterol and blood pressure, but also staggering weight loss – and they looked and felt so much better too.

The problem with red meat

The average Briton consumes 70g of red meat per day, with one in three of us consuming more than 100g per day. The WHO warns that eating just 50g of processed meat per day (less than half a burger or half a hot dog) increases the risk of bowel cancer by 18 per cent. It also warns that evidence shows that eating 100g of fresh red meat per day is associated with a 17 per cent increased risk of cancer.

A compound called haem, part of haemoglobin (found in the blood), is what gives red meat its colour. It might, however, also damage the lining of the bowel. This is because it's broken down in the gut by a family of chemicals called N-nitroso compounds, which have been found to damage the cells that line the bowel, causing other cells to have to replicate more in order to heal. This increases the chance of errors developing in the cells' DNA, which is the first step towards cancers developing and greatly increases the risk of cancer.

Medical research has found clear links between the consumption of red meat and the development of colorectal, pancreatic and prostate cancers. Other chemical constituents that occur naturally in red meat include nitrates and nitrites. Once ingested, they can be converted to cancer-causing compounds. That's why processed meat (such as bacon, sausages, hot dogs, ham, salami and pepperoni) are even worse – the troublesome nitrates and nitrites present in fresh red meat are added in significant quantities to these meats as preservatives.

Red meat and disease risk

I've seen first-hand that people whose diets are high in red meat have significantly higher health risks, not just of cancer, but also of heart disease, high blood pressure, diabetes and many other chronic diseases (such as gout). Heavy meat consumption has also been linked to depression, loss of mental concentration and dementia. Meat is also one of the biggest factors behind the obesity epidemic, as it is closely correlated with weight gain. According to the American Agriculture Department, Americans consumed 41 per cent more meat in 2000 than they did in 1950, and unsurprisingly, they're fatter and unhealthier than ever.

Research shows that animal protein, specifically in the form of red meat, might significantly increase the risk of premature mortality from all causes, including cancer, cardiovascular disease and type-2 diabetes. Women who eat more red meat have also been shown to have a greater risk of breast cancer, with an increased risk of 22 per cent among those who eat red and/or processed meat.

The diets of the longest-lived people

More convincing evidence is presented in Dan Buettner's bestselling book, *The Blue Zones*. People living in areas of the world identified as having the highest concentration of centenarians in the world (the so-called 'Blue Zones') live on a predominantly plant-based diet. Such populations include the Sardinians, for example, who eat meat around once a week, and the people of Okinawa, Japan, who get only 7 per cent of their calories from protein (the majority comes from sweet potatoes). So a small amount of meat might be beneficial for people who choose to eat it, but *moderation* is definitely the key here.

Plants and the gut microbiome

High red meat consumption has also been shown to increase the risk of colorectal cancer in both men and women. The mechanism is most likely due to an altered microbiome, the collection of microbes that live in your gut and play a key role in your risk of diseases such as cancer, obesity and diabetes.

As mentioned, high red meat intake is also associated with being overweight, and being overweight is a known risk factor for several cancers, including bowel, breast and kidney cancers. Although red meat might be high in protein, iron and zinc, it is devoid of fibre and other nutrients (found in abundance in plant-based proteins) that have a protective effect against cancer. Studies have also shown that people who eat a lot of red meat tend to eat fewer plant-based foods, which are protective against cancer.

Animal protein, especially in the form of red meat, also increases IGF-1, an insulin-like growth hormone that causes chronic inflammation, an underlying factor in many chronic diseases. Red meat is additionally high in Neu5Gc, a tumour-forming sugar that is linked to chronic inflammation and an increased risk of cancer.

Even the act of cooking red meat might increase your risk of cancer. When you grill or pan-fry meat, it can release heterocyclic amines and polycyclic aromatic hydrocarbons, substances that are known to cause cancer in animals.

High-meat vs high-plant diets

Low-carbohydrate, high animal-protein diets, which so many people are foolishly advocating these days, promote heart disease via mechanisms other than just their effects on cholesterol levels. Even if saturated fat apparently doesn't directly cause increased blood cholesterol levels, it doesn't mean that it doesn't indirectly cause heart disease via other mechanisms. Arterial blockages might be caused by animal protein-induced increases in free fatty acids and insulin levels, and decreased production of endothelial progenitor cells, which help to keep the arteries clean and healthy.

Dr Garth Davis, a leading bariatric (weight-loss) surgeon, head of a thriving weight-loss practice in the USA and author of *Proteinaholic*, says meat consumption, not carbohydrates, is a chief cause of obesity and diabetes in US society. The EPIC (European Prospective Investigation into Cancer and Nutrition) study, which followed 512,000 people in 10 countries for 12 years, concluded that meat, especially processed meat, is significantly associated with the development of type-2 diabetes, while fruit and vegetable consumption is associated with a decrease in diabetes development. This is just one such example. Study after study has shown that people eating fruit and vegetables, and especially grains, exhibit remarkably low levels of inflammation, and have considerably lower levels of diabetes than the general population. There is also a great deal of research showing that the more animal protein and saturated fat people eat, the more at risk they are of developing high blood pressure, and that meat eaters suffer more heart disease. Dr Davis quotes a study by the University of Copenhagen that implicated saturated fat (highest in red meat) as having 'a causative role' in heart disease.

Meat consumption also increases oestrogen levels, causing an adverse 'oestrogen dominance'. Women who eat more red meat, and fewer vegetables, have been shown to be more at risk of developing endometriosis, a chronic condition in which tissue that normally grows inside the uterus, grows outside it, often leading to severe pelvic pain and problems with fertility. As mentioned, high meat consumption is also associated with less fibre consumption, which serves to raise bad oestrogens and encourage the growth of harmful bacteria in your microbiome.

In addition, eating red meat increases uric acid and creatinine levels, thereby increasing your risk of kidney problems and gout. It also increases levels of hs-CRP, a marker of inflammation, and GGT, a marker of liver damage, so cutting it out will do your liver the world of good.

In case all that isn't enough to put you off, meat can be contaminated with superbugs, which can easily cause food-borne illness. Cooking reduces, but does not eliminate, the potential for exposure to disease-growth promoters in ground beef. And although you might have heard that 'grass fed is better', it's still not great. Data is still lacking to show that grass-fed meat is better for your risk of cancer, oestrogen levels and weight gain.

Reducing red meat for a longer life

A recent 2016 scientific study has found that cutting down on red meat can lead to a longer life and prevent early death. The research indicated that a 3 per cent increase in calories from plant proteins – found in vegetables, pulses, grains, nuts and seeds – can reduce the risk of premature death by 10 per cent. The results added further evidence that the consumption of red and processed meats was linked to higher mortality. The study of 130,000 people found that the risk of death from heart disease fell by 12 per cent if there was a 3 per cent increase in the amount of plant proteins in the diet. Replacing processed red meat with plant protein was linked to a 34 per cent lower risk of death from all causes for every 3 percentage points of calorie intake – certainly evidence in favour of The Food Effect Diet Vegan.

Cutting out red meat – a key to healthy weight loss

Countless studies have shown that most men and women lose weight when they switch to eating more plant-based foods instead of red meat. One study that followed 1,730 male employees for 7 years found that the more animal protein and saturated fats people ate, the more at risk they were of becoming overweight or obese. Given that around 65 per cent of British adults are overweight or obese, reducing your intake of energy-dense fatty meats seems sensible. Too much animal protein, specifically in the form of red meat, can also cause bloating, which no amount of crunches will get rid of. Meat is also extremely difficult to digest and disrupts intestinal bacteria, which leads to weight gain.

Some 'experts' might advocate low-carb, high-protein diets, but the science shows that this is completely the wrong way to be healthy. You might lose weight in the short term, but, I assure you, you will put it all back on.

Scientific studies aside, this is something I've witnessed myself among all my clients who used to eat red meat regularly: they all lose weight once they cut it out and switch to more plant-based proteins, even if they eat more carbohydrates than they were previously. This is my first-hand evidence in favour of The Food Effect lifestyle and approach. Not only do my initial 'meat and potatoes' clients come to me out of shape and overweight, but they also feel tired and sluggish, have stomach and digestive problems of all sorts, and lack the energy necessary to live an active, fulfilling life. Once they adopt The Food Effect approach to eating, they tell me that they've 'never felt more alive', and that they're no longer even tempted by a big fat juicy steak or burger.

If anyone is worried how they will get enough protein and iron without meat, just consider that the world's strongest primate, the gorilla, consumes enough of these nutrients by just eating fruit and vegetables and leaves (many green vegetables comprise 20–45 per cent protein), and, unlike the gorilla, you'll be eating plenty of plant-based sources of protein (nuts, beans, tofu, legumes, and so on), as well as vegan-friendly dairy and meat alternatives, so you definitely don't have anything to worry about.

As the author Michael Pollan famously said: 'Eat food. Not too much. Mostly plants.' It seems there is enough good research to support this, too. As you work through The Food Effect Diet Vegan programme, you can rest assured that it's designed not just to keep you slim, but also to optimise your health and prevent disease.

Cutting out red meat and following the options in both phases of The Food Effect Diet Vegan will not only ensure that you lose the weight you've always wanted to lose and keep it off, but, if you are one of the many people facing a lifetime on medication for what are termed 'lifestyle diseases', it can reduce the need for these, thereby transforming your life.

CHAPTER 6

The Facts about Fats

Don't go fat-free – choose healthy fats instead

Entire books and countless studies have been written about dietary fats. While you definitely don't need to know all the intricacies about fats to eat healthily, lose weight, stay slim and look and feel your best, there are definitely some basics that are worth knowing. Don't go fat-free – choose healthy fats instead.

Good fats should not be feared

As described in Chapter 2, one of my top tips for healthy eating and weight loss is to eat healthy fats and not try to go fat-free. You need some good fat to burn fat. This means eating healthy unsaturated fats of the type found in nuts, peanut butter, avocados, olive oil and various other healthy oils. These are included (in specified amounts) in The Food Effect Diet Vegan, as they are proven to lower the risk of heart disease and aid the body in the absorption of vitamins and minerals. Incorporating good fats into your diet helps to reduce sugar cravings, increase energy levels and keep you fuller for longer. Although too much fat can cause weight gain, too little of the right fats prevents your cells from functioning properly, which affects fat metabolism, hormone balance and energy – all leading to weight gain. That's why 'eat good fats' is one of The Food Effect Diet Vegan rules, and 'avoid trans fats' is another. Trans fats are often listed under the names 'hydrogenated' or 'partially hydrogenated' vegetable oil or 'vegetable shortening', and are found in many processed foods. They are toxic and have no health benefits whatsoever (more on them later in this chapter).

Fats are a great source of energy and provide vital nutrients for the body. Additionally, they help the body absorb nutrients, such as vitamins and minerals from vegetables and salads, more efficiently. Some nutrients, such as vitamins A, D, E and K, and carotenoids (antioxidants found in many fruit and vegetables), require dietary fat for absorption. That's why The Food Effect Diet Vegan meal options always have some healthy fat included in them – whether it be in the form of avocado, a little olive oil, nuts, seeds, tahini or hummus. They're all designed to maximise the nutrition in your meal, without racking up the calories; however, even with all their health benefits, fats are the most calorie dense of all the macronutrients (containing 9 calories per gram, compared to 4 calories per gram for carbohydrates and protein), so you do have to be mindful of your portion sizes. Just because they're healthy, it doesn't mean that you can eat them freely, or that they can't make you gain weight. Even if you stick to consuming only healthy fats, you still have to watch your portion sizes and quantities when consuming foods such as nuts, hummus, tahini, avocado and olive oil (that is, all the things marked with an asterisk in the tables on pages 31–2). There's definitely benefit in consuming a little olive oil, but, as mentioned previously, consuming it in excess will lead to the consumption of too many calories followed by weight gain. The same goes for nuts – learn what a normal serving size looks like (based on the portions specified in the meal plans) and stick to that.

Luckily for you, there's no guesswork involved. Whether it's avocados, nuts, peanut butter, or even seeds on your porridge,

I've done all the hard work for you and, as long as you stick to my suggestions in the meal options, you'll always be consuming exactly the right amount of fat to provide you with the optimum health benefits, without compromising your weight-loss goals.

Fats: the basics

The four main types of fat found in foods are saturated fats, monounsaturated fats, polyunsaturated fats and trans fats.

Saturated fats

There are several types of saturated fats and are typified by the white fat you see marbled through red meat or on the underside of poultry skin. Thankfully, it's easy to avoid saturated fat being vegan, as it's mainly found in animal products. It's fine to consume small amounts of saturated fat, but excess amounts can promote raised cholesterol levels. Coconut oil is an exception to this rule, due to its unique molecular structure. It can help the body burn fat and lower cholesterol (more on this below). In general, The Food Effect Diet Vegan avoids large quantities of saturated fats.

Unsaturated fats

Monounsaturated and polyunsaturated fats are generally what I am referring to when I talk about healthy fats. Foods that fall into this category include avocados, nuts, nut butters, seeds (such as pumpkin and sunflower seeds), chia seeds and olive oil. These are loaded with nutrients and have been shown to help with weight loss, keep you satiated and give you glowing skin. Omega-3 fats are the best known of this group of beneficial fats, and are found in chia seeds, pumpkin seeds, walnuts and linseeds (also known as flaxseeds). On top of their endless health benefits, omega-3s have been found to increase a hormone called leptin, which helps to promote satiety and banish unnecessary cravings, so embrace those omegas.

Trans fats

Completely artificial and manufactured trans fats are what we really need to watch out for and avoid at all costs, as I've said earlier. These fats are usually created in a laboratory and are solid at room temperature. They are therefore useful to the food industry and are also popular with fast-food restaurants, as they are cheap and long lasting. They are found in things such as vegan margarine, cakes, biscuits, pastries and fast foods such as chips. They've been linked to cancer, heart disease and diabetes, over and above weight gain and obesity. They've been shown to raise (bad) LDL cholesterol, and lower (good) HDL cholesterol, as well as blocking the absorption of good fats. It's for these reasons that foods containing these fats are listed in the 'Stay away' column in the tables in Chapter 2. They do nothing to benefit your health, weight or well-being. Avoid them altogether.

Specific fats

Here is some essential information on the benefits and uses of specific fats.

Coconut oil

Coconut has an endless array of health properties that have been shown to benefit the heart, brain and digestive system due to its unique healthy fat content, antibacterial effects and balance of dietary fibre, protein, antioxidants, vitamins and minerals. The rich source of healthy fats – medium-chain triglycerides (MCTs) – found in coconut flesh and oil, has been shown to help lower the risk of heart disease by increasing healthy (HDL) cholesterol without raising unhealthy (LDL) cholesterol. These wondrous MCTs also help with weight management, by reducing appetite, boosting metabolism and increasing the activity of fat-burning cells.

Coconut oil is brilliant for cooking due to its high smoke point. This means that it is more stable, and less easily damaged and chemically altered when heated to high temperatures, compared with other oils, such as extra-virgin olive oil. The latter is super-healthy, but it is better for drizzling and dressings than for heating and cooking. Although coconut oil is a saturated fat, it's a unique kind, and one I'm in favour of (unlike those from animal-based foods), and it is allowed in moderation on The Food Effect Diet Vegan.

Extra-virgin olive oil

This contains more healthy monounsaturated fatty acids than any other natural oil, plus a small amount of iron and a good level of vitamin E, a super-antioxidant. One compound found in olive oil, a monounsaturated fatty acid called oleic acid, is an anti-inflammatory and has also been shown to prevent certain cancers. The downside of extra-virgin olive oil is that it has a relatively low smoke point, so that its flavour and some of its nutritious properties start to degrade at high heats. It's best used in dressings and on salads; however, light refined olive oil (not extra-virgin) is safe to heat and use for roasting, cooking and frying. It possesses many of the same health benefits as extra-virgin olive oil.

Avocado oil

Cold-pressed extra-virgin avocado oil is one of the healthiest culinary oils available. This extremely versatile, healthful and nutrient-dense fruit oil is 100 per cent natural, and, like olive oil, is high in vitamin E and monounsaturated fatty acids including oleic acid. It has a very high smoke point of 255°C, making it stable at high temperatures and thus perfect for everything from cooking and sizzling, to drizzling and dipping.

Sesame oil

Although sesame oil has far fewer minerals and vitamins than olive oil, it does have good polyunsaturated fat levels, so it provides some healthy omega-3 fatty acids. It has a smoke point similar to that of coconut oil, and can be heated to 200°C without any negative effect. It has a bold flavour that best complements Asian and stir-fry dishes. Use sesame oil sparingly due to its rich flavour and high calorie count.

Nut oils

Of the most popular nut oils, walnut oil is rich in heart-healthy omega-3 fatty acids, and hazelnut oil is rich in vitamin E. Unfortunately, heat alters their taste, and they can taste burnt very quickly. They are best drizzled on salads or added to vegetables.

Nuts

Nuts have long been feared as the enemy of weight loss due to their high calorie count – but, thankfully, the truth has now largely won out and people are finally coming to their senses about these glorious little wonders, realising that eating nuts does not make you fat. In fact, it's quite the opposite; not only have studies shown that those who consume nuts are slimmer, but their endless health benefits (ranging from improved heart health to glowing skin) are now also undisputed. Here's the lowdown on these little nutritional powerhouses.

Good for health

Countless scientific studies have shown that eating nuts can really boost your health and prevent illness – most notably, improving general heart health and specifically lowering the risk of heart disease. And the benefits don't end there. A review of 25 scientific studies (what's known as a meta-analysis study) led scientists to conclude that eating 70g of nuts per day resulted in lower total cholesterol and lower 'bad' LDL cholesterol. Ironically, it's their high polyunsaturated and monounsaturated fats that lower cholesterol levels in the blood.

Other studies suggest that eating just a handful of nuts each day might help to reduce not only heart disease and high cholesterol, but also high blood pressure, high blood-sugar levels and excess abdominal fat (which is know as metabolic syndrome).

Good for staying slim

Many people think that because nuts are high in calories, they'll inevitably pile on the pounds; however, research shows quite the opposite to be the case. One Spanish study of almost 9,000 adults showed that those who ate nuts at least twice a week had a much lower risk of gaining weight over the next few years compared with those who rarely or never ate them. Another study found that despite having the same calorie intake, adults who included 84g of almonds in their daily diet in place of some of the carbs, had around a 60 per cent greater reduction in weight and body fat after six months compared to those who did not eat them.

The bottom line: not only does eating nuts not cause weight gain, but it might actually help you to lose weight (and stay slim).

Good for training and fitness

Nuts contain the perfect combination of protein, to protect muscle tissue and repair damaged cells, and healthy essential fatty acids, which have incredible anti-inflammatory properties. Consuming some protein before and – especially – after a workout has been shown to have beneficial effects. A small amount of pre-exercise protein increases amino acid levels during exercise, which serves as a biochemical signal that tells muscles not to break down protein for fuel. After exercise, consuming protein reduces the negative effects of muscle damage on your ability to exercise the next day. As mentioned, the essential fats found in all nuts will further protect your muscles against free-radical damage both during and after training, by strengthening muscle-cell membranes.

The practical bit

Nuts are portable, versatile, nutritious and delicious. If you're looking for the easiest healthy snack to stash in your handbag, briefcase, pocket or office drawer, nuts fit the bill. They are the perfect food to grab for an instant energy boost during that dreaded mid-afternoon slump. Because of their ideal combination of protein, healthy fats, fibre and low-GI carbs, they promote satiety and prevent you reaching for unhealthy sugar- and fat-laden junk food. Keeping your hunger in check between meals not only keeps your energy levels stable throughout the day, it's also an indispensable weight-loss strategy.

Each nut has its own specific nutrient profile and health benefits, but any nut will offer heart-healthy fats, vitamin E (a critical antioxidant), fibre, protein and a host of other beneficial nutrients. Any nut is a great choice, as long as you stick to the portions listed below, as well as those laid out in The Food Effect Diet Vegan meal plans.

Although all the evidence is in favour of nuts for healthy weight control, you definitely can't go eating a whole big bag each day (I discuss this in more detail on page 109). Keep portions to around 30g per day (or as specified in snack options), and ideally stick to unsalted varieties. If you're out and about or buying for work or travelling, buy nuts in pre-portioned bags (weighing 30–50g), or do your own portioning at home, into small snack bags or Tupperware containers, once you've bought a big bag.

The numbers of nuts that make up a 30g portion are roughly: 24 almonds, 18 cashew nuts, 28 peanuts, 14 walnuts and 49 pistachio nuts. Note that portion sizes might be smaller if specified with fruit in your Food Effect Diet Vegan meal plan and options.

Avocados

As well as being extremely delicious, these are a wonderful source of the healthy monounsaturated fats, which have been shown to help lower blood pressure and are extremely good for your heart. They have been shown to improve 'bad' LDL cholesterol and reduce the risk of heart disease in people who are overweight and obese. They are also a rich source of fibre, which helps to control blood-sugar levels, and potassium, which is good for lowering blood pressure.

Although it's commonly known that bananas are a source of potassium, avocados contain even more of this essential nutrient. Half an avocado contains more potassium than a medium-sized banana, so you won't even be missing out, as bananas are a no-no on The Food Effect diet, as explained on page 55.

Avocados have also been shown to help people feel fuller for longer and stave off the munchies between lunch and dinner. A recent study in *Nutrition Journal* found that overweight adults who ate half an avocado at lunch had a 40 per cent decrease in the desire to eat again over the next three hours – and, for some, the feeling of fullness lasted a whole five hours. Because avocados are so creamy, they also help to satisfy cravings.

Guacamole (made from avocados) is a great option when you're craving a high-fat treat. Avocados also contribute towards strengthening your immune system, being rich in glutathione – a powerful antioxidant, detoxifier and free-radical scavenger.

Lastly, but certainly not least importantly, avocados help to keep your skin, nails and hair healthy, strong and glowing.

Losing weight while looking and feeling your best

The Food Effect Diet Vegan approach to fats and diet in general is not just aimed at weight loss, but it is also targeted at improving overall health, including heart health and disease prevention. It is backed up by the latest research, which shows that consuming plenty of vegetables, nuts and olive oil is more effective than using drugs such as statins in treating heart disease. A diet rich in fruit, vegetables and healthy fats such as olive oil, nuts, seeds and avocadoes, has long been known to be good for the heart, and the latest studies confirm this. Those who ate mainly along Mediterranean lines (higher in monounsaturated fats, and low in saturated fats such as those from meat and butter) were 37 per cent less likely to die during the study than those who ate a diet heavier in saturated fats, and that was after adjusting for age, sex, class and exercise.

Simple signs that suggest you might be lacking in essential fats are dry skin, constipation, poor wound healing, frequent infections, inflammation of the joints, and small bumps on the backs of your upper arms. You might be saying goodbye to many of these problems once you start eating The Food Effect Diet Vegan way.

As you can see, The Food Effect Diet Vegan encourages you to eat from a wide variety of healthy fat sources, while reducing/ eliminating saturated and trans fats, for both health optimisation and weight-loss reasons. All the good fats are included in the correct amounts in the meal plans. You certainly won't be going fat-free with The Food Effect Diet Vegan, but you'll be relying on the healthiest choices of fats, thereby promoting weight loss and keeping you full and satiated.

CHAPTER 7

Snacking and Overeating

Banish cravings, avoid overeating and master your self-control

In Chapter 2 you read the fundamentals of The Food Effect Diet Vegan way of life and The Food Effect Diet Vegan rules. These will help to ensure that you eat healthily, minimise hunger and cravings, and keep your blood-sugar levels stable to achieve your goal weight and maintain your health and weight over the long term; however, even with a practical, easy-to-follow meal plan and manageable set of rules, there will still be times when you feel that you just 'need' that bar of chocolate, or want to eat way more than you should.

Although I do see the occasional client who never gets cravings or the urge to overeat, this is certainly not the norm. Although I can assure you that The Food Effect Diet Vegan will leave you feeling more satisfied and less deprived than other diets out there, I know that having a few additional tactics – both practical and psychological – will go a long way in helping you to banish cravings, avoid overeating and master your self-control.

Why do we overeat?

We've all overeaten at some point (if you never have, you're an admirable and rare human being). It can happen for a range of reasons: boredom (shown to be one of the most common reasons), loneliness, sadness, stress, anxiety and access to large volumes of tempting food, to name just a few. If you overeat only very occasionally, for example at a festive meal or party, and you are then able to take control and get back on track with your healthy-eating plan the next day, that's quite normal and won't be a major issue in your weight-loss journey.

Unfortunately, far too many of us overeat on a regular (if not daily) basis and are gaining weight, or not losing it, as a result. If you regularly go to bed bursting with food, or finish a meal feeling uncomfortably full, now might be the time to take a closer look at why you are overeating and develop ways to control it.

Overeating on a regular basis is often strongly linked to our mood. Stress, sadness, frustration or any unresolved emotion can cause you to turn to food for comfort. This behavioural response might have been taught to us by parents or carers who have offered food, usually of the sweet, sugary type, to soothe us when we were a crying injured infant or a sad teen, for example. Or it might be self-taught – we remember the pleasure that we instantly experience when we eat certain foods (think of your favourite vegan dessert or tub of ice-cream), then we seek out this sensation again to ease emotional pain. Unfortunately, although food does temporarily numb emotional pain or fill an emotional void, the pain or void is not fixed, so the habit of overeating might continue for days, weeks and months, if not years, while we continue to reinforce this short-term reward system that we have developed. Additionally, it is not difficult to overeat. The fullness mechanism in the body is nowhere near as tightly regulated as hunger is. It's far easier to override your fullness signal, especially when high-calorie, high-fat and high-sugar food is readily available, than it is to ignore your hunger signals for a significant amount of time.

Being aware of when overeating is most likely to occur for you in your day-to-day life is a crucial part of taking control of overeating, as is learning to listen to your body when it comes to the volume of food it needs. If you have been overeating for a long period of time, this might be especially difficult to just stop doing naturally on your own. That's why The Food Effect Diet Vegan Attack Phase and Lifestyle Phase meal plans and options have been designed and laid out with all portions specified for you. All you have to do is follow them, and I can guarantee you won't be overeating.

How to take control

1. **Know your high-risk situations** These are different for each person. You might overeat socially, or perhaps only in private; you might do it during that mid-afternoon slump; or you might not be able to control late-night cravings even after you've had dinner. Whatever the case might be, the chances are that there is a specific time or situation when you are most likely to overeat. Once you identify which times are risky for you, it's simple to develop strategies to manage these situations (see more on this in the tips to control cravings and avoid overeating on page 107). Focus on implementing these strategies at the times you are most vulnerable. You might find that you need to have your mid-afternoon snack close to the time you are heading out to dinner so that you don't overeat when you're out at a restaurant, or have a cut-off time for stopping to eat in the evening if late-night snacking is your problem. Whatever your high-risk overeating time is, the key is to implement some management strategies for it then.

2. **Get in tune with your hunger and fullness signals** Many of us eat so much or so often (or both), that we can't even remember the last time we felt really, truly hungry. I'm not suggesting that you should let yourself reach the point of feeling starving (in fact, it is a Food Effect rule that you do not do this), but if you can't recognise true hunger, it's also difficult to gauge when you are actually full. For many of us, it might only be at the point at which we feel stuffed or uncomfortable. If this is the case, try paying closer attention to the point at which you start to feel full and satisfied. Usually, it's a mouthful or two before the actual full feeling, especially as it takes the stomach at least 10–20 minutes to register true fullness, and even longer for the food you eat to reach the end of your intestine where more satiety hormones are released. Give it some time before deciding that you need seconds. Chew each mouthful slowly, and put your cutlery down between mouthfuls. This will help you to gauge how your body is feeling so that you won't eat like a machine on autopilot – and, as I said earlier, eating slowly will also ensure that your brain actually registers when you've eaten enough food, before it's too late.

3. **Tailor your environment** Quite simply, if it's not there, you won't eat it. If you keep a steady supply of tempting treats at home or at work, it's quite natural that when you're feeling bored, tired, stressed or down, you'll eat them. Keep away from the pile of sweets, crisps, biscuits or birthday cake that colleagues bring to work. Although, of course, it's amazing that vegan food has become so much more widely available recently, it also means that many tempting treats (biscuits, cakes, doughnuts) are now vegan-friendly, so you need as much willpower and discipline as anyone else. If you tell yourself that those things are off-limits for you (they are all in the 'Stay away' column, see pages 32–4, after all, and for good reason), you won't be caught in the

overindulgence trap. Once you start with those foods, they just trigger cravings for more unhealthy, sugary or fatty foods, so it's easier not to start eating them in the first place.

4. **Learn to compensate** Although, ideally, none of us would ever overeat or overindulge from now on, that's highly unlikely and also unnecessary – after all, what's life without some pizza or ice cream! One strategy for when you do overindulge is to compensate. By this I definitely don't mean starving yourself the next day or even skipping a meal, but, as discussed in The Food Effect Vegan Lifestyle Chapter 12, you might want to choose a salad or soup (or any of the options in the Attack Phase plan, Chapter 11) for a meal, rather than a vegan burger in a bun with sweet potato wedges or a large vegan pasta dish – even though those things are allowed in the Lifestyle Phase once you're on to that, after the first four weeks. Learning to compensate healthily will help you to feel physically better when you have overeaten and help balance your overall intake so that the occasional indulgence doesn't hamper your weight-loss goals.

Top tips to control cravings and avoid overeating

Here are a few simple strategies to banish those cravings and avoid unnecessary overeating or snacking.

1. **Avoid your triggers** You crave what you eat, so change what you're eating to the right foods (see the 'Eat this' options in Chapter 2) to weaken your cravings for the bad stuff. As I've said, the foods in the 'Stay away' columns in Chapter 2 are labelled 'Stay away' for good reasons: they do nothing to benefit your health or weight, or to help banish cravings.

2.   **If you don't want to eat it, don't keep it in the house.**

3.   **Put leftovers away immediately.**

4.   **Avoid buffet and 'all-you-can-eat' restaurants**, especially if you find this type of scenario tempting; this is just a sure-fire ticket to overeating unnecessarily.

5.   **Allow yourself to indulge within limits** Practise portion control or a healthier indulgence in moderation (such as a few squares of good-quality dark chocolate, or a decadent vegan dessert made with healthy ingredients . . . yes, such things do exist). See the snacks and sweet treat recipes on pages 265–75 for ideas.

6.   **Plan ahead** If you know there's an upcoming situation where you are going to indulge, allocate calories and factor them into your eating plan that day (but don't go there hungry – you'll just set yourself up for disaster). My best advice would be: when you do go for a treat and allow yourself to indulge, make it pleasurable by choosing something you truly enjoy, and savour every bite.

7.   **Schedule snacking** If you find yourself constantly tempted to have that bag of crisps and eventually feel so hungry that you can't resist it, make sure that you never skip lunch or your mid-afternoon snack, and try to schedule it before the time you get ravenous. So if, say, by 4.30pm you feel ravenous every day, tell yourself that on any given day 3.30pm is your snack time. Buy a healthy snack ahead of time or have something with you (at work or in your bag) so that you don't get the urge to go out and buy that giant bag of crisps.

8. **Focus on protein and fibre for a filling snack** There's nothing wrong with having a snack in between meals: in fact it's encouraged and specified in The Food Effect Diet Vegan rules and meal plans, even during the Attack Phase. Our bodies typically need something to eat about every 3–4 hours. For the most satiating and energy-boosting snacks, choose options that contain both protein and fibre; for example, an apple with a tablespoon of peanut butter or a handful of almonds, or hummus with carrot sticks. There is a long list of options in the menu plans on pages 199–202, so you don't need to think too much about this one – it's all there for you. Adding more fibre and protein to your snacks slows digestion and ensures better blood-sugar regulation, making you less likely to reach for unhealthy snacks and junk food.

9. **Go nuts (in moderation)** If, despite having eaten enough, you still have a strong urge to snack, drink two glasses of water and eat a 30g serving of nuts (around 12 walnuts, 18 cashew nuts, 20 almonds, 28 peanuts or 49 pistachio nuts), then reassess how you feel. Nuts are my all-time favourite snack, which I recommend to clients, as they fulfil the criteria of the tip above (they contain protein and fibre) in one neat package. Nuts are packed with an amazing profile of healthy fats, fibre, protein and micronutrients (vitamins and minerals), while satisfying hunger cravings. If you're out and about and suddenly feel ravenous between meals, bags of nuts are a staple in many food shops and make an extremely healthy choice. They are far better than crisps, sweets or sugar-laden chocolate. A single serving of nuts contains only about 130 calories, but beware of those jumbo-sized bags that can contain a whopping ten servings. One solution is to pack your own nuts as single servings in a small snack bag or sealable container. One serving of nuts is about 30g, but remember that the number of pieces varies by nut, as specified above. Pistachio nuts are a great choice

because not only are they lower in calories than other nuts, but also cracking each one open takes time, allowing you to enjoy them for longer.

10. **Sip something steamy** If you're craving something sweet, or if your stomach is rumbling mid-morning or afternoon and there's no healthy food in sight, try a hot almond milk or soya milk latte instead. Caffeine in moderation has health benefits (or you can go for decaffeinated), and you'll be getting calcium, protein (if you use soya milk), vitamins and minerals from the milk (most plant-based milks used in coffee shops are fortified), while avoiding all the calories, sugar and unhealthy fats found in vegan sweets, biscuits and processed snacks. Herbal teas are another great option for any time of the day – there are many delicious sweet flavours on the market that are perfect for a mid-morning or mid-afternoon pick-me-up, as well as in the late evening when the munchies strike.

11. **Stay well hydrated** You've heard this one before but it deserves reiteration. Drink, drink, drink. And by this I mean water. Often when we think we're hungry, we're actually just thirsty, so make sure you drink plenty of water throughout the day, as well as 1–2 glasses before every meal or snack you have. Symptoms of dehydration can mimic the feelings of hunger, so before you reach for a 250-calorie vegan chocolate or granola bar, drink a bottle of zero-calorie water. Water aids weight loss by helping your kidneys to flush out excess toxins and chemicals, which might be slowing down your metabolism. If you have difficulty drinking enough plain water – which should be around 2 litres a day – herbal teas, green tea and lemon in hot water are all just as good.

12. **If you're eating due to tiredness, take a power nap instead.**

13. **Brush your teeth and gargle with mouthwash** if you're inclined to eat unnecessarily, especially late at night. You'll be less likely to go and eat more food with clean teeth and the taste of mint on your tongue.

14. **Distract yourself and let stress go using other techniques** We all tend to snack when we are bored, so find other ways to stay busy. Keep occupied around the house, or even take up a new hobby. Taking your mind off food will help to reduce unnecessary mindless snacking. Read a book or file some papers to keep your hands and mind busy, or take a walk after dinner. Cravings usually last around ten minutes, so find a non-food-related activity to pass the time and take your mind off food. Bored? Call a friend, read a magazine or a good book, or do some tidying or organising. Angry? Try to do some exercise to get rid of the anger in a way that empowers rather than disempowers you. The burst of activity will also release endorphins (feel-good hormones) that make you feel happy and less stressed. If you can hold off from craving-induced eating for ten minutes, you might well overcome the urge altogether.

15. **Dodge the comfort food trap** This is especially pertinent when winter comes around. It's tempting to curl up on the sofa and binge on stodgy carbs and sweet treats, but far from making you feel good, typical so-called comfort food can leave you feeling tired, lethargic and moody. Instead, get your sweet fix from fruit or any of The Food Effect Energy Balls or healthy sweet treats (see Chapter 13), which raise your serotonin levels naturally.

16. **Get your soup on** When you crave comfort food, heat up a large bowl of soup made with lots of vegetables and beans. It's flavourful, hearty, high in satiating protein,

fibre and nutrition, and low in fat and calories – the perfect thing to keep you feeling full and satisfied (see the soup recipes on pages 253–60).

Snacking staples

Stock up on the healthy vegan snacking staples listed below (and refer to the list of snack options in The Food Effect Diet Vegan meal plans and options). Make sure you have these foods on hand at home or at work to avoid the urge to seek out an unhealthy sugary chocolate bar or a bag of crisps instead.

Raw vegetables

Crunchy vegetables can help to ease stress and cravings in a purely mechanical way. Munching celery or carrot sticks can ward off tension by helping to release a clenched jaw. Whenever you feel the urge to snack, but you know you've eaten enough and just want something to munch on, chew on some carrot or celery sticks. Keep a jar or container full of them submerged in cold water, for a refreshing crunchy snack. When you're looking for something a bit more substantial, pair your chosen raw veg with a serving of hummus.

Fresh fruit

Fresh fruit never fails. You can't go wrong snacking on fruit, such as disease-fighting blueberries, apples and oranges, which have been shown to reduce the risk of heart disease and certain cancers. Additionally, the potassium, magnesium and calcium in most fresh produce have been proven to help lower blood pressure. Ready-cut fresh fruit and fruit salads are sold in most food shops and supermarkets – perfect for when you're on the go and in need of a sweet fix. Berries are a particularly good option, as they are very low in calories and sugar, yet their sweetness helps to replace sugar cravings and leaves you feeling fresh and satisfied.

Dark chocolate

Thankfully, there are many great vegan dark chocolates on the market. This type of chocolate contains two compounds that can lower stress levels: anandamide, which binds to receptors in the brain that produce feelings of euphoria, and phenylethylamine (PEA), a substance naturally found in the nervous system that is released throughout the brain when we fall in love. If you fancy a sweet treat, dark chocolate (anything that is at least 70 per cent cocoa) is sure to satisfy your cravings and has also been shown to protect against cardiovascular disease and help to lower blood pressure. It is far better than other sweet snacks that contain large amounts of refined sugars, which deplete the B vitamins that are needed for energy and leave you feeling unsatisfied and in need of more sweet sugary foods. The flavonols found in cocoa – the main constituent of dark chocolate – also improve circulation and increase blood flow to the brain, which helps you think and see more clearly. Luckily for vegans, non-dairy dark chocolate actually contains the highest amount of powerful antioxidants compared to milk chocolate. Limit your portion size to two to four squares a day for a snack. See the meal plans for portions and specified options incorporating dark chocolate.

Oatcakes

Because oats are so high in fibre, few things take longer for your stomach to digest, allowing a sustained release of the feel-good neurotransmitter serotonin. Oats, in the form of porridge, are therefore included as part of your breakfast options, but oatcakes make a great snacking choice, too (as specified in the snack options). Studies have shown that including five servings of whole grains a day as part of a calorie-controlled diet can help you to lose abdominal fat and lower your levels of C-reactive protein (CRP), a predictor of heart disease, stroke and diabetes. Many brands of oatcakes are now vegan-friendly (such as Nairn's).

Fortified unsweetened almond milk and other calcium-rich foods

Including calcium-rich foods, such as unsweetened almond milk or soya natural yoghurts (both of which are fortified with calcium), as part of a balanced diet, has been shown to aid weight loss (see Chapter 4). Additionally, 1,000mg of calcium a day will help you to maintain bone mass when trying to lose weight. Calcium can also reduce muscle spasms and soothe tension, and, in fact, fortified plant-based milks have the same amount of calcium as regular dairy milk. Calcium has also been shown to reduce stressful PMS symptoms, such as mood swings, anxiety and irritability, which all do nothing to help with emotional eating. An almond milk latte or a soya natural yoghurt using fortified plant-based products, therefore, make great calcium-rich snacks.

Chickpeas

As mentioned in the section on The Feed Effect Vegan favourite proteins (see Chapter 4), chickpeas are a fantastic source of fibre and protein, and have a low glycaemic index. This combination makes them particularly good at helping with weight management, as well as preventing cravings. In an Australian study, adults who ate 100g of chickpeas a day for four weeks, ate fewer processed snack foods and felt fuller, compared to those who didn't include chickpeas in their daily diet. One cup of cooked chickpeas provides 50 per cent of your daily fibre requirement, promoting long-lasting energy, satiety and good digestion, which all contribute to curbing appetite and cravings. Try my recipe for

Sweet-and-Spicy Crunchy Chickpeas for the perfect waistline-friendly, craving-busting snack (see page 265).

Hummus

As it's made from the aforementioned wondrous chickpeas, hummus makes the perfect healthy energy-boosting snack that is sure to satisfy any creamy–salty cravings. The addition of tahini also makes it rich in calcium (as well as protein and fibre), too. It's great paired with vegetables such as red peppers, carrots and cucumbers, or spread on to some Ryvita, brown rice cakes or oatcakes. Try my recipe for Best-Ever Healthy Homemade Hummus (on page 255), but there are many great, healthy, store-bought options if you're short of time.

Oranges

The magic nutrient here is vitamin C. A German study in the journal *Psychopharmacology* found that vitamin C helps to reduce stress and return blood pressure and cortisol back to normal levels following a stressful situation (raised cortisol is linked with weight gain and fat storage). Vitamin C is also well known for strengthening the immune system, and it helps with the absorption of iron. So next time you're feeling stressed out about something, go and peel yourself an orange!

Nuts

It is a shame that some people avoid nuts, as they are high in calories, because if eaten in the right amounts, they are definitely one of the best snacks out there. Nuts provide essential healthy fats and, in some cases, omega-3s, which are crucial for the brain, improve circulation and prevent inflammation. These will keep hunger at bay for several hours until your next meal. Snacking on nuts might help you to shed pounds and reduce abdominal fat. Researchers have found that people who ate almonds for six months as part of a calorie-controlled diet lost 18 per cent of their body weight compared to those who did not. Additionally, monounsaturated fats found in nuts have been shown to lower harmful LDL cholesterol levels, while increasing the good HDL cholesterol that benefits your body. All nuts are a great snack that can be portioned ahead of time for when you get hungry. Because nuts are calorific, make sure you measure your serving (see portion sizes on page 101). Although all nuts make a great snack, a few deserve a special mention:

Almonds are rich in B vitamins, which make you more resilient during bouts of stress, and vitamin E, which helps to bolster your immune system. To get the benefits, snack on about 20 almonds every day (or as specified in the snack options in Chapters 11 and 12). Another way to get your fix is to eat some almond butter – although make sure you stick to a small serving (1–2 tablespoons).

Pistachio nuts and walnuts Both these nuts will help to keep your heart from racing when things get stressful. Research has shown that eating a handful of pistachio nuts a day lowers blood pressure so that your heart doesn't have to work overtime. Walnuts have the most antioxidant power of all varieties of nut and are rich in magnesium and healthy omega-3 fatty acids (a great source for vegans). Walnuts have also been found to lower blood pressure, both when you are at rest and under stress. As well as making a great snack, chopped walnuts can be sprinkled over salads, cereal or porridge.

Avocados

One of the best ways to reduce high blood pressure is to consume enough potassium, and, as mentioned, avocados actually have more of this essential nutrient than bananas – half an avocado has more potassium than a medium-sized banana. The mono-unsaturated fats found in avocados also help to lower blood pressure, and are extremely heart healthy. Guacamole can be a great option when stress makes you crave a high-fat treat.

A word on visualisation

Visualising your future self can play a huge role in developing self-control with food. We've all been there before – opening the jar of peanut butter to have 'just one teaspoon', or that tub of Ben and Jerry's Non-Dairy Chocolate Fudge Brownie (yes, it exists) sitting in our freezer for 'just one scoop', but, before you know it, you're scraping the last remnant from the jar or have reached the bottom of the ice-cream tub.

The 'just one' mentality is about as difficult to master as the Rubik's Cube. When it comes to eating well (that is, sticking to the right foods and the right quantities), most people will admit that self-control is the hardest part. But here's the good news – science has cracked the code to impulse-proofing eating habits. Research from the University of Zurich postulates that being able to focus on your future needs is one way to achieve self-control. The researchers found that if you bypass your 'present self' to love your 'future self', you can resist that in-the-moment temptation (so it *is* possible to stop yourself from finishing that tub of ice-cream).

How do you fend off your self-indulgent urges and stay in touch with your future desires? Here are some of my tips for doing this:

- Put reminders of your health goals in plain sight to help you visualise the person you want to be. For example, you might want to write on a big Post-It note: 'I never feel good after over-indulging in junk food, and I don't want to be a person who always craves sugar', or 'Sugar makes me feel tired, lethargic and moody. I don't want it to be a staple part of my diet.'

- Keep your long-term achievement of health at the forefront of your mind by writing motivational notes and creating an inspiration board. You can do this by hand, having a board on Pinterest, or saving inspirational pictures and quotes on your phone and browsing through them regularly.

By doing the above, you'll create your own strong vision of your ideal healthy self (but remember: we are all different, and it's important to be realistic and not make unhealthy comparisons with others). When that tub of Ben and Jerry's Non-Dairy Chocolate Fudge Brownie seems a little too appealing, you can check back in with the needs of your 'future self' that you have pictured so strongly in your mind and find the strength to say 'No thanks, maybe some other time.'

CHAPTER 8

Dining Out Done Right

How to make eating out vegan healthy and enjoyable

People often assume that dining out and losing weight are incompatible, or, at best, very challenging, and with the addition of being vegan, you might worry that this is going to be extremely difficult. I've seen from my clients that going out to eat is probably the one thing that new vegans fear most, but the good news is the reality can be very different, and dining out can be an enjoyable, satisfying and delicious experience all while losing weight (or staying slim) on The Food Effect Diet Vegan.

Eating out in general has become so common in our culture these days. Restaurants were once mainly visited on special occasions, but now, according to the National Restaurant Association, almost half of adults eat at a restaurant or order a takeaway every day, for convenience, variety or taste. People are looking for fast, easy and tasty food to fit their busy lifestyles. Whether it's in sit-down restaurants, food courts, takeaways, office cafeterias or hospital canteens, dining out has become an integral part of everyday life, and with the rising popularity of veganism, there are now more and more vegan options available in most restaurants and food chains.

Thankfully, by following The Food Effect Diet Vegan rules and tips (laid out in this chapter) when dining out, you can still lose weight and maintain an active social life, while following a vegan lifestyle.

Although there are usually several healthy vegan options to choose from when dining out, there are still many more bad choices available (think deep-fried tofu and oily noodles), and a lot of opportunities to go wrong and ruin your waistline. This doesn't mean that you shouldn't eat out and that you need to become a social recluse just because you're leading a healthy life-style and watching your weight. The Food Effect approach is all about enjoying life and living normally. This diet is based on the approach I took in devising plans to suit incredibly busy people who don't have much time to spend preparing home-cooked meals in the kitchen. Eating out vegan can be healthy and enjoy-able; this chapter guides you on everything you need to know about dining out (or ordering in), done right. If you do prefer to cook and prepare your own meals, the recipes in Chapter 13 will give you everything you need.

Before getting on to specific types of food and restaurants, as well as tips for eating when travelling or at an airport, here are my general tips for eating healthfully when dining out.

Before you order

If you're nervous about maintaining your healthy-eating plan, or about there being healthy vegan options available, think ahead, do some research, and plan where you're going to eat or order in from. Check out the restaurant's website and consider what meal options are available. Look for restaurants or takeaway options with a wide range of menu items, and, of course, some healthy vegan choices. With so many places available, you don't need to go for that one Chinese option with only greasy, fried vegan food.

Plan ahead If you know you're going to be eating a large meal in the evening, consider your food choices for that entire day, not just that night. Perhaps have a slightly lighter breakfast and lunch. I definitely don't suggest that you skip meals or arrive at dinner starving (that goes against The Food Effect rules), but you might choose a healthy salad that day instead of a large hummus sandwich, for lunch for example.

If you are familiar with the menu, decide what to order before entering the restaurant. This tactic will help you to avoid any tempting foods that might not be particularly healthy.

If you are trying a new restaurant, take the time to look over the menu and make careful selections in order to avoid making unhealthy decisions. Some restaurant menus may have a special section for 'healthier' choices, or options such as whole-wheat pasta or brown rice for sushi.

Pay attention to restaurant menu terms for clues as to fat and calorie content. Baked, braised, broiled, grilled, roasted, poached and steamed all imply less fat and calories than battered, fried, creamed (for example with coconut cream and/or vegan margarine), crispy, sautéed and so on. Avoid or limit the latter choices as much as possible.

When you order

Stick to ordering baked, braised, broiled, grilled, poached, roasted or steamed foods, as mentioned above. This can apply to everything from tofu to dumplings, to vegetables and vegetable sushi.

In place of fries or chips, choose a side salad, steamed vegetables or a baked potato.

Order vegetable side dishes (or potatoes) baked, steamed, boiled or roasted rather than fried. For both weight loss and vegan reasons, ask the waiter to omit any butter, cream or creamy sauces. You can even stress that you're vegan to ensure that they don't use any of these whatsoever.

If you are ordering a soup, stick to broth-based soups such as minestrone or vegan noodle soups, or non-creamy vegetable soups, such as gazpacho.

Refer to the tables in Chapter 2, and stick to foods in the 'Eat this' (or 'Be careful') columns, avoiding anything that comes under 'Stay away'.

When choosing or assembling a salad, avoid items such as hard vegan cheeses (which are usually made of coconut oil and additives), creamy vegan dressings (unless specified as low fat or light) and croutons.

For salads, always order the dressing on the side so that you can control how much you use – and use it sparingly. Better yet, use a squeeze of lemon, balsamic or rice vinegar instead of a dressing. And, of course, you can add salt and black pepper.

Ask the waiter about ingredients or preparation methods for any dishes that you're unsure about. Being vegan actually makes this a lot easier, as you have good reason to do so. It's perfectly OK to make special requests, but try to keep them simple; for example, it's reasonable and sensible to ask for a baked potato or extra side salad in place of French fries, or for no mayonnaise or butter in your sandwich, and for sauces and dressings to be served on the side.

If you're getting a sandwich made up for you, boost the bulk and nutrition by adding tomato, lettuce, peppers, grated carrot or other vegetables. Choose protein-rich fillings such as chickpeas, hummus or vegan cream cheese (made with almond milk or cashew nuts) on whole-grain bread. Ask for mustard, ketchup or salsa (which are all allowed on The Food Effect Diet Vegan) and avoid butter, full-fat mayonnaise and margarine (for both vegan and weight-loss reasons).

During the meal

Avoid eating too much before your meal even arrives. That means no bread dipped in olive oil, crisps or cashew nuts – wait for your meal to be served instead. Once you get stuck into the bread basket it's not hard to eat two or three pieces before dinner, and that can equal a whole meal's worth of calories before you even get to your main course.

Avoid all-you-can-eat specials, buffets and unlimited salad bars, if you tend to eat too much at this type of meal. If you do choose a buffet, fill up on salads and vegetables first. Take no more than two trips and use a small plate.

Eat lower calorie foods first If everyone is ordering a starter, a vegetable-based soup or fresh salad is a good choice. Avoid anything deep-fried or battered. Follow it with a light main course.

Limit the amount of alcohol you drink to no more than one drink per evening out (more specifics on alcohol in Chapter 9).

Tempted by sweet, creamy vegan desserts? During your first four weeks on the Attack Phase these are a complete no-no. You may, however, order fresh fruit or fruit salad without whipped (vegan or coconut) cream or vegan ice cream. Another great trick is to drink more. By that I mean order a cup of (decaf) coffee or herbal tea at the end of the meal, so that you're occupied while the other diners are tucking into their tiramisu or hot chocolate cake. You'll be less tempted to eat dessert if you're busy sipping your mint tea and making good conversation. Once you're at the Lifestyle Phase, I'd still advise you to avoid calorific vegan desserts. If you must (and if the other diners agree), order one vegan-friendly dessert with enough forks for everyone at the table to have a bite. Alternatively, sorbet is not a bad choice – although it does contain sugar, it doesn't include fat, and it's not too high in calories.

Take home leftovers. If you can't finish your extra-large vegan sandwich or pasta dish, you don't need to eat it just to avoid wasting it: take half home for another meal or lunch the next day. Any restaurant will be more than happy to pack up your leftovers if you ask – that way you get two meals for the price of one and don't ruin your waistline.

Specific types of cuisine

Italian

As discussed earlier, owing to low-carb diet crazes, foods such as pasta and pizza have gained a bad reputation, and those looking to lose weight would usually never dream of touching these foods (and if they did, they would guiltily assume they had broken their diet). Yet in Italy, people eat pasta daily without the country having the same obesity rates as those in the UK and the USA, and on The Food Effect Diet Vegan you can certainly enjoy them too. Here's how.

Staying slim while enjoying pasta

My aim here is to bust a few myths. Pasta is not the weight-loss enemy it's often made out to be. There is every reason why you can eat this versatile carb without piling on the pounds (while gaining valuable nutritional benefits in the process). Here is the how and why.

When I suggest incorporating pasta into my clients' diets I am often met with an incredulous stare and the response: 'But isn't pasta fattening?' The truth is, I hate this question. No – pasta itself is not fattening. Pasta is a low-fat food with just 1.5g of fat per 75g serving. It's usually the specific type, how much you eat and what goes on your pasta that makes it a potential diet disaster (think big bowls of white pasta laden with thick cream sauce and melted cheese – even if it's vegan). I'm certainly not giving you free rein to eat all types of pasta in vast quantities, so here are some of The Food Effect rules and tips.

Rule 1: White pasta is out, whole-grain pasta is in (where possible). Whole grains (such as oats, barley and brown rice) contain fibre, protein, healthy fats and an abundance of vitamins and minerals. Good-quality whole-wheat pasta and brown rice pasta provide a good dose of these nutrients. There is also a variety of additional healthy pasta options available now, such as chickpea pasta and red lentil pasta. The fibre and protein in all these (non-white) pasta varieties means that a smaller portion will keep you fuller for longer, and ensure your blood-sugar levels remain stable. Whether you go for whole-wheat or brown rice pasta (which is gluten-free), both have several further benefits:

1. One serving of whole-wheat pasta (75g uncooked weight) provides about a quarter of your daily fibre requirements. As mentioned above, increased fibre helps you feel fuller (on fewer calories), thereby aiding and boosting weight loss.

2. Both whole-wheat and brown rice pasta are good sources of B vitamins such as thiamin (essential for energy production, carbohydrate metabolism and nerve-cell

function), riboflavin (needed for healthy skin turnover and maintenance), and niacin (needed in fat, cholesterol and carbohydrate metabolism, and the production of many body compounds, including sex and adrenal hormones).

3.   Pasta is one of the most versatile foods around, with countless available types (such as spaghetti, penne, fettuccine, tagliatelle, macaroni, ravioli and lasagne). With numerous ways to serve up pasta dishes (think added vegetables and sauces) you will never be stuck for options. It's also the perfect match for tomato sauces, which are rich in the super-antioxidant lycopene.

If there's no whole-wheat pasta on the menu, there's no need to avoid ordering pasta (unless you're on the Attack Phase, where pasta is out for four weeks), but make sure you stick to the next rule.

Rule 2: Be careful how much pasta you eat Although pasta itself is low in fat and nutritious, it does contain a reasonable amount of calories. This is not necessarily a bad thing, but it does need to be taken into account in determining how much to eat. A 75g serving (uncooked weight) provides around 270 calories. This is perfectly suitable for a main meal (with additions), but it's often hard to stop at just one serving, and the bowls you get in a restaurant usually contain at least two or three servings. Spaghetti as a main dish can weigh in at a whopping 1,000 calories – more than half your daily calorie allowance. A simple way to tackle this sensibly is to eat half and get the waiter to pack up the other half, or share a main-course portion with a friend or partner. Another good trick I often share with my clients is to fill half your bowl with vegetables – either fresh spinach or salad leaves, or steamed green beans or broccoli. This works because volume plays a large role in determining how satisfied we are from a meal. If we've had a large, full bowl of 'real' food, we'll feel just as satisfied even though half of it was low-calorie vegetables and the other half pasta.

Rule 3: Watch what goes on your pasta Thick, creamy sauces – even if totally vegan – are out. They are guaranteed to add hundreds of calories and grams of fat to a meal. Opt for tomato-based sauces wherever possible. I love nothing more than a bowl of spaghetti topped with a classic tomato sauce. If you're eating in a vegan restaurant (or at home), you can sprinkle nutritional yeast over, for a delicious healthy cheesy flavour and a ton of good nutrition. If you're eating in a non-vegan restaurant, it might be worth specifying 'no Parmesan' with your order, as they sometimes toss it on right at the end.

Staying slim while enjoying pizza

You probably never thought you'd hear a doctor or nutritionist tell you that pizza can actually make a healthy balanced meal, but I'm going to do just that. If you consider its components, pizza has the potential to pack in plenty of goodness. The base provides healthy carbohydrates, especially if it's whole-wheat flour, which is actually a good source of protein, fibre and other important nutrients, the tomato sauce provides high levels of the cancer-fighting antioxidant lycopene, plus endless other sources of nutrients if you load up your pizza with vegetable toppings such as red onion, peppers, mushroom and sweetcorn. With that kind of combination, the bad reputation given to pizza can be a thing of the past.

Of course, let's be honest here, a thick-crust, vegan-cheese laden pizza is far from a health food. Although this does vary, one slice of a large, thick-crust pizza contains 300–400 calories, and an average 16g of fat – 7g of which is saturated – as a result of the oil-glistening vegan cheese. But if you order carefully, there's no need to deprive yourself any longer. Here are some suggestions for ways in which you can enjoy a pizza while keeping the experience waistline friendly.

1. **Half please** Unless you're an active teenage boy or man, you generally only need half a pizza for a decent-sized meal (with a side salad or preceded by a vegetable soup). To prevent overeating and the excess calories that come along with it, either share a vegan pizza with a fellow diner, or take the other half home for later (because, let's be honest, who would ever turn down leftover pizza?). It can be reheated, or even enjoyed cold the next day.

2. **Stick to smart sides** They might be tasty, but side orders such as French fries and onion rings are loaded with calories and trans fats, as they are usually cooked in unhealthy vegetable oil. Keep your sides light, yet filling, by sticking to things like a side salad or cooked vegetables.

3. **Skip the vegan cheese** Eating a cheese-less vegetable pizza is an easy way to cut out a great deal of calories and unhealthy saturated fat. A good 'saucy' pizza topped with veggies is absolutely delicious and far from bland and boring, and it allows those delicious vegetables to take centre stage instead.

4. **Thin is in** Thin-crust pizza is far lower in carbs and calories than those deep-dish pizza pies. It's also far more authentic and Italian in style, so be sure to order thin crust wherever possible.

5. **Go whole-wheat** If available, order a whole-wheat crust. It's much higher in fibre and protein than white, so you feel fuller from less and your body won't turn it straight into sugars and fat. It'll also help to keep your blood-sugar levels stable and you feeling fuller for longer. If it's not an option,

a thin-crust pizza made with white flour, loaded with veg and tomato sauce, without cheese, is still a healthy and balanced option.

Yes, there'll always be those who are willing to order a salad while everyone else devours their pizza and who would never dream of touching a slice, but that's not the approach I advocate. Eating should be pleasurable and enjoyable – especially on occasions when you're dining out or ordering in.

Now that you know my pasta and pizza rules you can go ahead and enjoy these foods guilt-free, The Food Effect Diet Vegan way, and, rest assured, they will not cause you to pile on the pounds.

Chinese

Chinese food in the West caters to our taste for fried food and heavy, meat-based entrées, rather than the healthy grain and vegetable-based dishes traditionally found in China. Fortunately, being vegan does automatically eliminate a large proportion of these unhealthy options, but there are still plenty of unhealthy vegan-friendly Chinese options that will not aid your weight loss results (or make you feel good after eating them, either).

When choosing what to order in a Chinese restaurant, steer clear of deep-fried dishes such as vegetable spring rolls, deep-fried seaweed, fried rice and fried tofu (often battered or coated with a sesame crust), which all pack in thousands of calories and a whopping amount of unhealthy saturated fat. The oils they use in Chinese restaurants are far from healthy olive oil. Also avoid anything described as 'sweet and sour', as this ultimately means coated in a sugary sauce (and sometimes batter too) and fried. Stick to low-fat dishes that are stir-fried or steamed, and packed with vegetables and protein, if possible (such as steamed tofu). If steamed vegetables or rice seem bland, order a stir-fried vegetable dish and mix it with the steamed side dish (such as broccoli or green beans and mangetout). The sauce from the stir-fry adds flavour to the steamed food, while having a steamed option reduces the overall calorie and fat content provided by two stir-fried dishes together, without any compromise on taste. Noodle- and vegetable-based dishes are also a healthy and delicious option. If the noodles used are egg noodles, ask the waiter if they can substitute them for rice noodles to make it vegan-friendly – plus it's a super-healthy, low-calorie option too.

Japanese (sushi)

Nowadays, sushi is becoming available almost everywhere you turn – from Japanese restaurants to supermarkets, grocery stores to local bakeries. And there are a lot more vegan options on the menu. Although it can provide a delicious and filling meal, sushi can also be a diet disaster if the wrong choices are made. Many people assume that opting for sushi is a guaranteed healthy option; however, this is certainly not always the case.

I'm often asked by clients whether they can eat sushi, what they should order, how much, and so on. A sushi meal, comprising of, for example, one or two basic cucumber/avocado rolls, can weigh in at a measly 200–300 calories or, at the other end of the spectrum, top 1,000 calories – think deep-fried tempura rolls. Although, unfortunately, there's no simple answer, and it's difficult to give a set quantity, what you order and how much of it there is, is what makes the difference, as is the context in which it is being eaten (for example, as a starter or as your main meal). Healthwise, you need to know quite a bit when making your sushi choices, so before you order and get stuck in, bear in mind these simple vegan-friendly tips for eating sushi and staying slim.

1. **Power up with protein and healthy fats** When choosing sushi as your main meal, make sure you incorporate a decent amount of protein. This is definitely more challenging when

it comes to sushi for vegans, as all fish options are off-limits. It takes a bit more thought to ensure a balanced meal, but it's totally doable with The Food Effect Diet Vegan tips. Although a cucumber roll might seem like the diet-friendly option, and indeed it is low in calories, you need protein to provide satiety and sustenance to your meal. An easy way to do this is to order a portion of steamed edamame beans, which are an excellent source of protein (you can have them topped with sea salt) along with your vegan sushi rolls, or have a bowl of miso soup with cubes of tofu in it, another great source of protein. You could even ask the restaurant to add some extra tofu to your bowl. When choosing fillings for your sushi rolls, avocados are an excellent source of heart-healthy, skin-enhancing monounsaturated fats, but they are also higher in calories than other vegetables, so don't go overboard with them. Perhaps stick to one avocado roll, and one of another vegetable variety (such as cucumber, carrot, red pepper, baby corn, and so on) along with the above suggestions.

2. **Go light on the rice** The basic rolls, such as avocado and cucumber, are all good choices, but they do come with white sushi rice, which is high in calories and lower in nutritional value than brown rice. As it contains practically no fibre or protein, the calories quickly add up and become converted straight into simple sugars and fat. That doesn't mean, however, that white rice can't be incorporated into a healthy diet in the right way. My advice is to try to get brown rice sushi, which is becoming more widely available in shops and restaurants, wherever possible. This will provide your body with added fibre, protein and various other nutrients, such as B vitamins, so that a smaller serving of sushi will get you satiated sooner, and for longer, as well as providing your body with added healthy nutrition, which is especially important for vegans.

3. **Don't be tempted by tempura** Stay away from anything on the menu labelled as 'crunchy' or 'tempura', as this indicates that the rolls or vegetables inside are coated in batter and deep-fried. Forgo the extra calories and unhealthy fats by avoiding these dishes altogether.

    Another new vegan-friendly option that is popping up in sushi restaurant chains and often included in the vegan sushi meals is *inari* sushi. Inari sushi is made of sushi rice wrapped inside seasoned deep-fried tofu pockets called *inari age*. These are certainly far from waistline-friendly, so avoid this altogether. Inari in the sushi rolls itself is thin strips of deep-fried tofu; try to avoid this, but if there's just a tiny amount in the predominantly vegetable-based roll, it's fine to have in moderation.

4. **Know your portions** Although traditional sushi is a healthy food, it's still important to stick to proper portions if your aim is to eat light and stay slim. An average vegetable sushi roll (about six pieces) contains about 150–200 calories. If you consume three rolls, say for lunch, which is not difficult, this amounts to a lot of calories – even before taking any added sauces or side dishes into account. As a guide, a sensible sushi meal would consist of a portion of edamame beans (around 150 calories) and one to two basic rolls such as avocado or cucumber, or one roll of a bulkier variety (such as the Itsu veggie dragon roll).

5. **Be mindful** In the same vein, because sushi is cut into those little pieces that pop perfectly into your mouth, it makes every extra bite seem so harmless. It's definitely a moreish kind of food that's very easy to lose track of. This is especially true if you're sharing rolls with family or friends, or eating them standing at a cocktail party or a wedding reception, as opposed to ordering a takeaway meal or dining in a restaurant. A good strategy is to put all

the sushi you plan to eat on your plate before you tuck in, as this will prevent you from getting carried away. Also, make use of those chopsticks – they'll force you to eat more slowly.

Greek

Typical of the famed Mediterranean diet, Greek food is one of the world's healthiest cuisines. It's full of heart-healthy mono-unsaturated fats (found in olives and olive oil), fresh salads and delicious vegetables. Although there's plenty of goodness to be had when dining Greek-style, there are a lot of dishes incorporating dairy, cream sauces, yoghurt and butter (for example, brushed between layers of filo pastry). Most of those translate into a hefty amount of calories and fat, so, luckily, you won't be missing out by avoiding them. Good options for vegans are a Greek salad (minus the feta cheese, and ask for the dressing on the side), whole-wheat pitta with a few tablespoons of hummus, tahini or baba ghanoush (aubergine dip), olives, vegetable dolmades (cabbage or vine leaves stuffed with a delicious herb rice mixture), roasted potatoes (as long as they're not in a lot of oil), roasted aubergine, grilled veggies, and a grilled vegetable wrap. Just make sure to enjoy everything in moderation.

Middle Eastern

There are plenty of healthy options on the menu in Middle Eastern-style dining, but at the same time there is also plenty of room to go wrong. The breads and spreads are delicious, but they can pack in hundreds of unnecessary calories, so do be careful.

The option of getting falafel served in a laffa (thick white bread) or pitta bread sandwich with generous helpings of hummus and tahini, not to mention the trend of adding French fries to it, is far from waist-friendly. Skip the laffa or pitta and you'll save hundreds of calories. Thankfully, the things that are off-limits for vegans – *shawarma*, which is usually lamb or chicken, dripping in oil and fat, and has the skin included – are definitely not things you'll be missing out on, for vegan, health and weight-loss reasons. Far healthier are chickpea-based falafel balls. Although I do advise staying away from fried falafel balls in general (for example, when buying for home, especially as there are so many healthy baked falafel brands stocked in supermarkets now), when dining out occasionally, it's absolutely fine to have a portion of falafel. Get this on a plate with salads (Israeli salad is a great healthy choice) and/or vegetables. Some couscous or tabbouleh salad is also perfectly fine and healthy to have with your meal. Make sure you stick to non-fried options of veggies and salads, pickled vegetables, carrot salad or shredded cabbage salad, rather than going for calorie-laden deep-fried aubergine.

Indian

Traditional Indian dishes that feature a variety of vegetables, chickpeas, beans, lentils and rice are great for a low-GI, high-fibre, healthy, plant-based way of eating – exactly what The Food Effect Diet Vegan prescribes. A vegetable curry, lentil dhal or chana masala (chickpea curry) paired with some steamed basmati rice, makes a perfect, healthy meal. Alternatively, combine some tomato-based side dishes such as beans or chickpeas and vegetables in light (non-creamy) sauces with steamed basmati rice, for the perfect meal in both the Attack and Lifestyle Phases. Although The Food Effect approach always advocates brown rice over white, Indian basmati rice is an exception: although white, basmati rice is higher in protein and fibre than regular white rice, so you can enjoy it guilt-free (see box on page 53).

Indian food and many of the curries can be healthy, but there are definitely some things to avoid. Some vegan curries are made with large amounts of full-fat coconut milk or cream, so don't be too shy to ask the waiter how the dish is prepared. Avoid samosas (deep-fried pastries filled with vegetables), and if you choose to have some bread with your meal (and you certainly can once you are on the Lifestyle Phase), stick with baked breads such as naan (check that it is made without dairy yoghurt) or whole-wheat chapatti, and avoid any fried breads. Whatever you order, make sure to ask for no butter, ghee (clarified butter), cream, or paneer (cheese).

A final word on dining out

Remember that there's not a restaurant out there that demands you finish what's put in front of you. Think about the amount of food you've been served, the company you're with, and that you're also out to have a good time. Eat slowly, enjoy your food and don't be afraid to leave anything that seems excessive or not in line with The Food Effect Diet Vegan way of eating and living.

Healthy eating when travelling and at the airport

Whether you're taking off on a long-planned holiday, heading home or travelling for work, being on the road can wreak havoc on the best-laid eating plans. Travellers are often faced with a dilemma: either bring your own food, which takes some planning and foresight, or buy a meal or snack on the way to, or at, the airport, which might result in a limited selection and poor nutritional choices. Airports in particular can be a challenge: giant muffins, multipacks of unhealthy sweets and chocolates, fast-food restaurants and temptation galore. But travelling needn't ruin your weight-loss efforts. Follow the tips below for eating healthily when travelling and on the go.

Snack sensibly The processed snacks that are the mainstay of airport shops don't satisfy hunger for very long. Processed foods that are high in fat and refined sugar, such as crisps, vegan biscuits and sweets, are all digested very quickly, raise your blood-sugar levels rapidly, and actually promote hunger and cravings. Instead, go for nuts, as they are naturally filling, extremely healthy and contribute to stable blood-sugar levels (preventing further hunger and cravings). Bags of nuts are a staple at airport shops and, indeed, are a healthy vegan-friendly choice (refer to 'Eat this' in the tables in Chapter 2). Nuts are a great source of protein, fibre and heart-healthy fats, and a single 30g serving contains only about 150 calories. But, as mentioned previously, beware of those jumbo-sized bags that can contain a whopping ten servings and can easily add up to a whole day's worth of calories. Do your own portioning as single servings into small zipper bags or containers (see page 101) to pack into your hand luggage when travelling.

If this is impossible to do in advance, buy nuts in pre-portioned bags (30–50g) so that you don't overeat. Alternatively, pack some homemade energy balls (see the recipes in Chapter 13), any of which make the perfect, portable filling snack. They are quick and easy to make, and you can easily make a batch ahead of time and keep them in the freezer for when you'll be travelling or on the go.

Fresh fruit and vegetables never fail Fresh fruit or chopped vegetables with hummus make smart, filling, on-the-go snacks. Whole fresh fruit and ready-cut fruit salads are sold at many air-port shops, or you can easily pack an apple or two in your bag.

Beware of hidden ingredients Items that might seem healthy and are labelled 'suitable for vegans', for example a hummus and falafel wrap, are often loaded with excess oils, tahini and dressing, packing in more than 500 calories and 25g of fat per sandwich. Read the labels to check the ingredients and calories, and stick to sandwiches on wholemeal bread with vegetables and some healthy plant-based protein, such as chickpeas or a light serving of hummus, rather than processed vegan cheese.

Grab a coffee If healthy food is nowhere in sight and your stomach is rumbling, grab a tall almond milk or soya milk latte. The milk is full of calcium, vitamins (and protein, if soya milk) and is extremely filling and satisfying, especially if paired with some fresh fruit such as an apple. You can make it a decaf if you want to sleep during the flight.

Stay hydrated As we have seen, dehydration can make you feel tired and hungry, when actually you're really just thirsty. Water is nature's perfect thirst quencher and is totally calorie free. It also helps to keep your skin healthy and glowing, which is important, as travelling and plane journeys can do just the opposite.

As you can see from this chapter, awareness and a little thought are all that are needed to make healthy choices when dining out or travelling. No longer does being vegan and watching your weight mean that you are stuck at home having to eat a salad every night. From day one on The Food Effect Diet Vegan, you can enjoy eating out with family and friends, while sticking to the plan and losing weight.

CHAPTER 9

Raise Your Glass

Moderate alcohol consumption is part of the programme

Here's the part that you've been waiting for: can you drink alcohol on The Food Effect Diet Vegan? I have good news for you: the answer is yes, even from day one. During the first four weeks – the Attack Phase and therefore the strictest part of the diet – you are allowed up to three drinks per week. I discuss what that means and the best choices to make on pages 140–2. Once you have completed the first four weeks of the diet and are on to the Lifestyle Phase, you can have up to one drink (that is, a glass of alcohol) per evening (or the equivalent, seven drinks in total, per week).

Although it's true to say that heavy drinking is indeed unhealthy and is linked to heart and liver disease, as well as to an increased risk of various cancers, moderate drinking, which is what The Food Effect Diet Vegan allows, has been shown to be extremely beneficial for the heart and circulatory system, and might even protect against type-2 diabetes. Moderate drinking, if done wisely, will not compromise your weight-loss goals either. There are numerous studies showing that moderate alcohol consumption reduces the risk of obesity and weight gain. One study that followed more than 19,000 women for a period of nearly 13 years revealed that women who consumed one to two alcoholic beverages daily were at least 30 per cent less likely to gain weight than non-drinkers. In another 2004 study, conducted at the Harvard School of Public Health, researchers reported that one drink per day did not contribute to weight gain, especially in women. In fact, alcohol might increase metabolism slightly so that you actually burn more calories. Researchers have found that consuming alcohol after a meal increased the number of calories burnt after both high- and low-carbohydrate meals. This might help explain the finding of these researchers, and many others, that moderate drinkers have less body fat than abstainers.

More recently, research has increasingly suggested that moderate alcohol consumption does not represent a dietary risk factor for developing obesity. In fact, a study published in the *Archives of Internal Medicine* found that light to moderate drinkers gain less weight than teetotallers over time, and have a decreased chance of becoming overweight or obese. I've seen this myself, first-hand, with clients who consistently lose weight without abstaining from alcohol. In fact, a study from Finland that included a total of 24,604 randomly selected men and women aged 25–64 concluded that: 'A physically active lifestyle with abstention from smoking, moderate alcohol consumption, and consumption of healthy foods maximises the chances of having a normal weight.'

As already mentioned, most diets are temporary and people only stick to them for a certain period of time because they are too restrictive, and most diets make you cut out alcohol completely as well. Many people enjoy a glass of wine with dinner, or a drink with friends when out at the weekend, or with colleagues on an evening out after work. This is something many of my clients told me when they first came to see me, so to tell them to cut out alcohol altogether was simply not realistic (or I could have done so, but they wouldn't have listened). On top of that, feeling deprived over a long period of time sets you up for failure far more than a 100-calorie glass of wine does.

I knew that if people were to truly embrace The Food Effect as a lifestyle, moderate alcohol consumption had to be part of the programme. That doesn't mean that I shied away from advising people to cut back on their consumption, or that they always found it easy. When a busy trader, for example, came to see me looking to lose weight and get healthier, I advised him to cut down from three drinks after work every night, and even more at the weekend, to a maximum of one drink per night. It was a challenge, but if I'd told him that alcohol was not allowed at all, he would simply have given up on The Food Effect diet altogether. Being teetotal simply wouldn't fit into the social aspect of his corporate lifestyle. Acknowledging this was an important factor that I kept in mind in creating The Food Effect diet, and it's another reason why it is so doable and successful.

To help you decide what to order at the bar without compromising your weight-loss goals, here is The Food Effect Diet Vegan guide to alcohol (stick to the limits according to the two phases as specified above – three drinks per week during Phase 1; seven drinks per week in Phase 2). If you're strictly vegan, remember to check that your alcohol of choice is vegan-friendly, as non-vegan wines, for example, use finings made from fish to clear them.

DRINK THIS	BE CAREFUL	STAY AWAY
Bloody Mary	Beer	Alcopops
Champagne	Mimosa	Amaretto sour
Gin and diet tonic	Mojito	Cocktails mixed with energy drinks
Martini		
Red/white wine spritzer	Pina colada	Cocktails with cola mixers
Red wine	Rum and Diet Coke	Dairy-free creamy liqueurs

DRINK THIS	BE CAREFUL	STAY AWAY
Tequila	Vodka and cranberry juice	Frozen daiquiri
Vodka and soda water (plus lemon/lime)		Malibu and Coke/fruit juice
Vodka and diet tonic		Rum and Coke
Whisky		
White wine		

As with everything on The Food Effect Diet Vegan, the key is to make the right choices.

During the Attack Phase, make sure that your three drinks per week come from the 'Drink this' column in the table. During the Lifestyle Phase, try to stick to the 'Drink this' column, but if you occasionally choose a drink from the 'Be careful' list, that's also perfectly fine. Just ensure that you don't make those drinks your regular choice every night.

Throughout the Lifestyle Phase, try to avoid all the 'Stay away' drinks. Like the foods in the food tables listed in Chapter 2, they are in the 'Stay away' column for good reason: they do nothing to benefit your overall health and weight-loss goals and should be avoided, or enjoyed only on the very odd occasion.

Make sensible choices

Since you've now read that drinking in moderation is not unhealthy and will not cause weight gain (in fact, it might even help with weight loss), you will know that there's no need to give up alcohol. However, the key is to remain sensible and stick to the rules of moderation.

The UK Chief Medical Officer's guidelines for both men and

women is that to keep health risks from alcohol to a low level it is safest not to drink more than 14 units a week on a regular basis. The guidelines, which were updated in 2016, made the recommended limit the same for men as women. This equals six pints of average strength beer a week, which would mean a low risk of illnesses such as liver disease or cancer. The previous guidelines were 21 units for men and 14 units for women per week. An additional recommendation is not to save up the 14 units for one or two days, but to spread them over three or more days. This is exactly in line with The Food Effect guidelines for both phases of the diet.

For The Food Effect Diet Vegan I have also kept the rules the same for both men and women and allow three drinks per week during the four-week Attack Phase, and one drink per evening (or seven drinks per week) during the Lifestyle Phase. Note that if wine is your drink of choice, seven glasses a week will add up to more than 14 units (see the figures below). Try, therefore, to choose spirits on some nights, or if it's only wine you fancy, make sure to stick to six glasses a week maximum.

Alcohol – units and calories in brief

One standard alcoholic drink is:
- One small bottle (330ml) of regular (5 per cent) beer (1.6 units, 142 calories).
- A 175ml glass of (13 per cent) wine (2.3 units, 159 calories).
- A shot (25ml) of spirits (40 per cent) such as vodka, tequila or rum, either straight or in a mixed drink (1 unit, 61 calories, not including sugary mixes/soft drinks/fruit juice).

You also have to be mindful, especially once you're on the Lifestyle Phase, that you cannot have alcohol and that little bit extra of a vegan dessert or indulgent pasta meal for the week (as explained in Chapter 8). It's all about making choices and deciding which option you will enjoy indulging in more – the alcohol or the food. If you're dining out and fancy pasta with tomato sauce that night, you might want to lay off a second glass of red wine. If you're desperate to enjoy two glasses of alcohol one night, choose a leaner vegan main course, such as a vegetable stir-fry or salad with some plant-based protein, instead of the pasta.

Another thing to be cautious about is alcohol potentially putting you in an 'Oh, why not?' frame of mind that results in you eating or drinking too much. If drinking alcohol lowers your inhibitions to the extent that you wind up gorging on the contents of the bread basket or the salted bar snacks, then plan ahead and either make sure you've had a filling, satisfying meal or snack before you go out for drinks, or, if you're drinking while dining out, ask for a plate of vegetable crudités to snack on until your meal arrives. That dish of salted nuts can easily pack in several hundred calories before your meal even arrives. Also make sure you drink water between sips of alcohol to stay well hydrated and satisfied, and switch to water or sparkling water with lemon after you've had your one drink.

Remember why you enjoy having a drink in the first place: that is, to enjoy the time with friends, family or colleagues, not so that you can overindulge. There's no reason why alcohol should ever interfere with your healthy eating choices. You can have a great time, enjoy alcohol in moderation and make The Food Effect Diet Vegan work for you.

A few more tips

As you can see from the drinks table (page 140), your best bets for healthy low-calorie drinks are wine, champagne and spirits. If mixed drinks are more your thing, order less-caloric, lower sugar versions of your usual drink; for example, order rum and Diet Coke instead of rum and Coke. (Although I'm no advocate of drinking Diet Coke in general, in this instance it's far better for your health and weight than regular sugar-laden cola.) Or order vodka, tequila or other spirits with zero-calorie soda water and a splash of cranberry juice instead of a sugar-laden lemonade. Or, you could take a cue from continental Europeans and have a wine spritzer, that is half wine, half soda water. Do beware of sugary cocktails such as margaritas, Long Island iced teas and pina coladas, which can set you back anywhere from 400 to 650 calories – that's more than a McDonald's Veggie Burger. Opt instead for tequila on the rocks with a splash of lime cordial or juice, or vodka mixed with soda water and cranberry juice.

If you're out at a special event or social situation where everyone is ordering cocktails at the bar, either stick to one of the above, if possible, or have just one cocktail, then switch to water or sparkling water garnished with lemon or lime. I can assure you that no one will be any the wiser – so you won't seem like a party pooper, and you won't derail your health and weight-loss goals either.

CHAPTER 10

Exercise and Supplements

Stop stressing about the gym – it's all about what you eat

Relying on exercise for weight loss is a major mistake that many people make because they've been led to believe that it plays a big part in achieving great results. Whereas keeping active definitely plays a part in a sustainable weight-loss regime, it is certainly not the major part of it. You can exercise all you like, but if you are eating a bad diet full of unhealthy fats, sugar and processed foods you are unlikely to see any results. As any personal trainer will tell you: 'Abs are made in the kitchen', and 'You can't out-train a bad diet.'

The scientific facts back this up. In the past 30 years as obesity has rocketed, there has been little change (that is, no significant decline) in the physical activity levels in Western populations. This places the blame for our expanding waistlines solely on the type and amount of calories consumed.

There are many people out there who think that it is OK to eat a packet of biscuits, a big piece of cake or big slab of unhealthy chocolate because they will go for a run straight afterwards. This is no way to lose weight and achieve the results you want. In fact, you're putting in all that effort for nothing. The key to weight loss is what goes in your mouth. If you feel like eating a piece of cake or a vegan biscuit, go ahead and have one. But know that you've strayed from The Food Effect way of eating and might not lose weight that day. That's normal and OK, on the odd occasion. But don't get into the habit of eating badly and thinking you can exercise it off. It simply doesn't work and will leave you feeling dejected and upset at the lack of positive results.

Enjoy exercise for health, but watch your food intake for weight loss

Although I definitely advocate some form of exercise (even if it's just walking) on most days, I don't encourage my clients or those adopting The Food Effect lifestyle to spend a huge amount of time on exercise that they don't enjoy, or to have an unhealthy focus on it, as it is not the key to (or even a large part of) weight loss. Weight loss requires patience, effort and dedication to eating well. Excess weight is not something you can simply run off in the park. It might take a while (by that I mean several weeks, not years), but if done correctly, staying slim and in shape can be sustainable for your entire life. Don't make yourself miserable in pursuit of a quick fix by driving yourself crazy over exercise – it really isn't worth it and doesn't work either.

In an editorial published in the *British Journal of Sports Medicine*, three leading international health experts said that it was time to 'bust the myth' about exercise. They concluded that while physical activity was a key part of staving off diseases such as diabetes, heart disease and dementia, its impact on tackling obesity was minimal, hence public-health messages should squarely focus on unhealthy eating rather than exercise. The experts also pointed to evidence from the *Lancet* global burden of disease programme, which shows that unhealthy eating was linked to more ill-health than physical inactivity, alcohol and smoking combined. They blamed the food industry, with its advertising and celebrity endorsements, for encouraging the belief that exercise could counteract the impact of unhealthy eating. 'An obese person does not need to do one iota of exercise to lose weight; they just need to eat less. My biggest concern is that the messaging that is coming to the public suggests you can eat what you like as long as you exercise,' said leading London cardiologist Dr Aseem Malhotra. 'That is unscientific and wrong. You cannot outrun a bad diet.'

The Food Effect approach is directly in line with what these experts recommend. Countless overweight clients have come to me, having been misinformed that if they want to lose weight they need to exercise intensely every day. They believed that in order to be slim they had to 'kill themselves' at the gym or take up running, even if they didn't enjoy it. Many had been training rigorously with a personal trainer for months, getting up early for boot camps that they loathed, or spending almost every day in the gym (despite not enjoying it) for the sole purpose of losing weight, but the pounds had not shifted. These despondent, over-exercised clients all arrived at my practice overweight, frustrated and desperate – quite understandably.

On changing their diets (and, with many clients, even exercising less), the pounds dropped off. I had one client who, during our initial phone call before starting on The Food Effect, told me, 'My biggest problem is that I don't have time to exercise, so I can't lose weight.' I reassured him that he didn't need to do an iota of exercise (I'm not saying that's the ideal for health, but weight-loss-wise it would make no difference), and if he changed the way he ate, he could lose weight. Sure enough, David never took on any exercise, followed The Food Effect programme and lost 19kg (42lb), reaching his goal weight in just six months – all without any exercise or ever going hungry.

Why exercise doesn't result in weight loss

Now that we've established that exercise isn't as useful for weight loss as you might have been led to believe, I'll briefly explain the science behind why this is the case.

1. **It increases appetite** Although you might not feel hungry immediately after a workout, you'll definitely notice that on the days you've exercised your appetite increases later in the day. If you've ever been swimming or had an intense morning workout, you'll probably have noticed that you get ravenous later in the day. Often, you end up eating more calories on those days than you actually burnt off, because your hunger is so much greater. On top of increased appetite, exercising makes your body crave high-calorie foods to replace the lost energy from intense workouts, making it that much more difficult to resist a post-workout binge.

2. **Exercise doesn't burn that many calories** Unfortunately, exercise doesn't burn as many calories as we'd like it to. It's much easier to resist a small 250-calorie pack of Skittles (they're vegan), than to burn 250 calories on a treadmill. Unless you're doing triathlon training, exercise will probably only burn around 10 per cent of your energy intake per day. When you consider that your appetite increases and that exercise makes you crave high-calorie foods, it's even harder to achieve any significant calorie deficit.

3. **We overestimate how hard we have trained** Because exercise can feel strenuous and exhausting, it's common to think that you've burnt more calories than you have. People generally overestimate how many calories they've burnt, while underestimating how much they eat.

4. **Our bodies adapt** The human body is highly intelligent. When you exercise a lot and often, your body becomes more efficient at storing calories, and you end up burning fewer of them. This is known as 'metabolic compensation'.

5. **Exercise can increase cortisol and promote fat storage** Although exercise does increase metabolism, when you push yourself too much it can have the opposite effect and prevent weight loss. Pushing ourselves to do long runs, for example, can cause the body to release the stress hormone cortisol to keep us going, yet this hormone also encourages fat storage around the middle.

6. **We can begin to resent exercise** As I've witnessed first-hand through many clients, when you think you need to exercise to lose weight and you don't see the number on the scales dropping, you become resentful and begin to resent exercise. This can sabotage your relationship with physical activity, which should be something enjoyable and part of maintaining good health, not viewed as a chore and a punishment carried out solely in a misguided attempt to lose weight.

If exercise won't help with weight loss, why should you do it?

I've told you that exercise is not the key to weight loss, and I have described the science behind why this is the case; however, you do need to do some physical activity for the sake of your health and general wellbeing. Here are some things it is certainly beneficial for. Exercise:

1. **Boosts your mood** Exercise is proven to boost mood, and can even help to counteract stress and anxiety and

ward off depression. Exercise releases mood-boosting endorphins and helps to release stress, making you feel noticeably happier after physical activity.

2. **Helps concentration** and makes you smarter. Even a short ten-minute workout (such as one taken from a YouTube video), or a brisk walk outdoors, will instantly boost your concentration and aid cognitive performance. One study even showed that exercise can make you smarter by helping to grow new brain cells (a process called neurogenesis) and that your brain actually gets bigger.

3. **Increases your lifespan** The same study outlined above revealed that exercise has a beneficial effect on your genes, helping to reverse the ageing process at a cellular level.

4. **Lowers your blood pressure,** thereby reducing the risk of heart attacks and stroke.

5. **Increases bone density,** so that there is less risk of osteoporosis and fractures.

6. **Improves balance,** so that there is less risk of falls and fractures.

7. **Increases strength, flexibility and stamina.**

8. **Helps improve sleep.**

9. **Increases libido** and boosts your sex life.

10. **Gives you more energy** for both work and play.

What sort of exercise should you do?

Exercise doesn't need to be complicated. To gain all the health benefits of exercise listed opposite, you don't have to join a gym, hire a personal trainer or sign up for a marathon. My advice is simply to do what you enjoy, make it as enjoyable as you can and do it regularly.

If you're currently not doing much exercise, or any at all, try walking or some light exercise for at least 10–20 minutes every day (this can include your walks to work, the train, between public transport, and so on). This is not only good for your bones, body and circulation, but it also gives you time to think, breathe and de-stress – all of which are essential to a healthy lifestyle. Light exercise also helps to lower the stress hormones cortisol and adrenaline, high levels of which can be responsible for excess weight storage (especially abdominal fat, as explained earlier). On top of your light daily walking, try working out (anything that raises your heart rate) for either 10 minutes five to six times a week, or 20 minutes three times a week – you don't have to kill yourself to become fit and toned. You'll notice a difference in how you look and feel simply by adopting that.

If you do already love to exercise, and are doing more than that, that's fantastic and I'm obviously not going to tell you to stop. A study in the *American Journal of Clinical Nutrition* showed that those who see exercise as part of their lifestyle, rather than as a way to change their appearance, are most successful at keeping the weight off.

Supplements for vegans – everything you need to know

Supplements are a major topic in the health-and-fitness world right now, and a subject on which I'm often asked for my advice and opinion. The spectrum of supplements available today is so overwhelming, and there are more and more being created and targeted at vegans, making things even more confusing. What should you take, and when? Ask some people and you'll get an endless list that would cost you a small fortune.

I'm normally of the belief that most of us can get everything we need from a colourful, varied and balanced diet. This does, however, require more thought, planning and effort for vegans, as certain essential nutrients (such as vitamin B12) are much more present in animal-based foods, and others (such as iron), are much more easily absorbed from animal-based sources than the plant-based foods in which they're found.

The good news is that if you follow The Food Effect Diet Vegan meal plan and options in this book, the thought and planning has all been done for you. Everything has been carefully designed to ensure overall nutritional balance (on both a macronutrient and micronutrient level), and to include foods that are high in nutrients that are commonly lacking in a vegan diet; for example, vitamin B12 (found in fortified plant-based milks, fortified soya yoghurts, fortified nutritional yeast and breakfast cereals – all included in The Food Effect Diet Vegan options), calcium (found in fortified plant-based milks and yoghurts, dark green leafy vegetables, tahini, almonds, hummus and sesame seeds), and omega-3 fatty acids (found in walnuts, pumpkin seeds, chia seeds and flaxseeds).

I've designed the meal plan and recipes with all this in mind; however, the meal plan and options are all flexible and interchangeable (as you'll read in Chapters 11 and 12), and people tend to stick to the foods they like best and might not always vary things. There's no need to stress about potentially lacking certain vital nutrients, however, as I do advise all vegans to take iron, vitamin B12 and iodine (in one multivitamin) and omega-3, and potentially calcium and zinc depending on your diet and physical needs. Vitamin D is the one supplement I strongly advise everyone, whether vegan or non-vegan, to take (more on this below).

For ease, I'd recommend taking a good multivitamin that contains iron, vitamin B12, vitamin D, iodine and zinc (calcium is not usually included in iron-containing multivitamins, as they are not absorbed well together, so, if needed, this will be taken separately) and an omega-3 supplement separately (you can buy a vegan version, as omega-3 supplements are usually made from fish oil). Omega-3 is important for everyone, as it is crucial for brain functioning, heart health and overall health. It also has anti-inflammatory properties, which help to protect against insulin resistance, diabetes, heart disease and many other illnesses. You can meet your needs by consuming enough chia seeds, walnuts, pumpkin seeds and flaxseeds (all included in The Food Effect Diet Vegan meal plan and recipes); however, for ease, and if you aren't eating these foods regularly, I would advise taking an omega-3 supplement.

As mentioned earlier in the book, any plant-based milk you use should be fortified with calcium to ensure your calcium needs are met. If you don't tend to consume much fortified milk (or fortified soya yoghurts) and/or if you are a woman, it's worth considering taking a calcium supplement, for bone strength and protection (as women are more at risk of developing osteoporosis than men, and they only lay down bone density until the age of 25).

Lastly, I am a massive believer in the importance of gut health, and would recommend taking a good probiotic. The Food Effect Diet Vegan has been designed to optimise your gut health, being high in fibre and healthy plant-based whole foods, but low in sugar, refined carbohydrates and processed foods; however, there has been so much recent scientific evidence to highlight the importance of having good gut bacteria for all aspects of health, weight management, improved digestion and boosting immunity – even improved mood and preventing depression – that I advise taking a probiotic as well, although it's definitely not essential.

If you are confused about which supplements to take (brands, dose, and so on) I'd always advise discussing your own personal supplement needs with a qualified doctor and/or nutritionist.

Don't be D-ficient

As I've already mentioned, while I'm not one for advocating an array of unnecessary supplements and vitamins, there is one vitamin that I've always advocated, and I tell all my clients – men, women and children, vegans, vegetarians and meat eaters alike – to take, and that's vitamin D.

This 'sunshine vitamin' has recently become the rising star of the supplement world (finally) due to research suggesting that it does far more than just protect against soft bones and rickets.

Low levels of this vitamin have been associated with increased fat storage, among many other health problems, and the sad reality for those of us living in the UK is that we are definitely lacking in some good old sunshine.

Levels of vitamin D deficiency in the UK are the highest in 50 years, with one in five people suffering severe deficiency. The incidence of infant rickets, the bone-weakening condition that was rife in the Victorian slums, was at a record high in 2017 and 2018. Experts have attributed the problem to modern indoor lifestyles, the increased use of sunscreen, poor diet and cool summers.

Although vitamin D might be best known for promoting healthy bone growth, in fact most organs require (and therefore have receptors for) vitamin D. We now know that low levels (which are virtually guaranteed during the winter in everyone in the UK), are associated with an increased risk of conditions ranging from heart disease, multiple sclerosis and Alzheimer's disease to diabetes, breast cancer and bowel cancer. Even a mild-to-moderate deficiency can, in the long term, result in osteoporosis, making fractures more likely to occur in a fall.

A recent 2019 study looking at data from ten randomised control trials of supplements found that taking vitamin D supplements reduces the risk of dying from cancer by 13 per cent.

Additionally, as mentioned above, vitamin D levels have an impact on weight. Vitamin D deficiency causes the brain to issue hunger-signalling hormones, tempting you to reach for the biscuits and crisps. Calcium-rich diets have also been found to aid weight loss, but vitamin D is required to regulate calcium absorption. Therefore, you should definitely take a vitamin D supplement from October to March, if not all year round. Most of us have a deficiency of vitamin D in the summer as well, so keeping our levels up in the winter is crucial.

Although vitamin D is found in vegan foods such as fortified plant-based milks and breakfast cereals, it's virtually impossible to get an adequate amount through diet alone, even for non-vegans who eat salmon and eggs, the two major food sources of this vitamin. They would need to consume ten whole eggs to reach the required 10mcg per day. And, of course, on a vegan diet this is impossible and no amount of fortified almond milk will meet your needs.

The body depends mainly on internal production through the action of sunlight on the skin – which unfortunately we do not get enough of in the UK. Even if you live in a hot country, unless you sit out and sunbathe daily, it's unlikely that you will get enough of this vitamin through sunlight alone.

UK guidelines previously only recommend routine supplementation for those most at risk of deficiency (the elderly, pregnant and breastfeeding women, and so on); however, my advice to all would be to take a standard dose vitamin D supplement, which can be found in pharmacies and health-food stores, every day (1,000 IU per day). Thankfully, new national guidelines from Public Health England are now in line with what I recommend; as of 2016 their advice is that all Britons should consider taking a daily supplement of vitamin D, particularly from October to March. Doctors (myself included) welcomed this guidance, saying that vitamin D deficiency could be eliminated entirely with supplements costing an average of just £10 to £15 a year.

Exercise and supplements: tips to get you started

After reading this chapter, hopefully you'll understand why exercise is not the key to weight loss, and that the main factor in losing weight and staying slim is what goes in your mouth; however, there are far too many health and lifestyle benefits of exercise not to make it part of your routine. Here are some tips to help you as you begin The Food Effect Diet Vegan way of life.

- Check with your doctor first. If you are severely overweight or have any serious medical conditions, it is advisable to get your doctor's approval before embarking on any exercise programme.
- Choose activities that you enjoy. If you're having fun and enjoying yourself, even if you're working hard, you're more likely to stick to a routine.
- Set aside a regular time for exercise. Whether you sign up to an exercise class or decide to wake up a little earlier every day to do some exercise, scheduling it in as you would a work meeting will guarantee that nothing gets in the way of your good intentions.
- Partner up with a friend, family member or your partner. This makes it more fun and will increase motivation and commitment to your new fitness regime.
- Vary your exercise. There is no 'best' or 'right' exercise, just what works best for you. It's never easy, especially at the start, but once you begin to feel better, and have more energy and a new zest for life, you'll never want to give it up.
- Make sure to take a good multivitamin containing iron, vitamin B12, vitamin D, iodine and zinc, as well as an omega-3 supplement suitable for vegans.
- Women (and men) should consider a calcium supplement as well, depending on your diet and risk of decreased bone density.

- Consider taking a good probiotic for gut health and digestion.
- I'd advise discussing particular supplements (recommended brands, doses, and so on) and your own personal supplement needs with a qualified doctor and/or nutritionist.

CHAPTER 11

Phase 1, Kick-Start Your Weight Loss

The Food Effect Diet Vegan Attack Phase and meal options

This phase is all about kick-starting your weight loss and helping to banish cravings for good. It's the strictest phase of the diet, but you'll still be eating plenty (including carbs at every meal and dark chocolate on most days). It lasts for four weeks – just 28 days – which is long enough to completely resolve any insulin resistance brought about by eating too many unhealthy, processed carbs and foods.

Phase 1 is not low carb – it's about eating the right amount of the right carbs. You aren't, however, allowed things such as whole-wheat pasta or breakfast cereals during this phase, but you can reintroduce them (exact details are specified in the Lifestyle meal options in Chapter 12) once you reach The Food Effect Diet Vegan Lifestyle Phase.

The meal plan is designed to allow ample portions of healthy vegan proteins, good fats, vegetables, fruit and low-GI carbs needed for optimum satisfaction and blood-sugar stability. This includes low-GI fruit (such as apples, pears, oranges and berries) and starchy vegetables (such as sweet potato), where portions are specified. There is no benefit in cutting these out – they contribute fibre, important nutrients (especially necessary for a vegan diet), vitamins and minerals, and heart-healthy antioxidants. Most salads and vegetables (including all green vegetables, carrots, tomatoes, broccoli, cauliflower and butternut squash) are unlimited (as long as they're not in any oil). The proteins come from a wide range of sources, so you can be flexible. If you don't eat tofu, for example, you can substitute it with another specified protein source, such as tinned chickpeas, lentils or kidney beans, a vegan burger or baked falafel balls.

By the time this phase ends, any unhealthy cravings you have for sweets, chocolate, baked goods and unhealthy starches will essentially have vanished. Even though this is the strictest phase, you will by no means be going hungry. You'll be eating three substantial meals, plus two satisfying snacks (including a post-dinner/late-evening treat) a day, so you'll certainly never feel deprived.

The meal plan is laid out day by day for ease and simplicity, but you can interchange any of the options within the same meal category on any given day – that is, you can switch the specified breakfast for any of the breakfasts from any of the days, and the same for lunches and dinners. You can't interchange a lunch for a dinner, however: you can only interchange meals and snacks that are within the same categories. In short, as long as you consume no more than a specified breakfast, lunch, dinner and two snacks on each given day for 28 days, you'll lose weight (about 6–12lb in the first four weeks alone, although, as previously mentioned, this will depend on how much weight you have to lose, because the more excess weight you're carrying, the more you can expect to lose).

The Attack Phase rules

Keep moving (light activity, as long as you're not sedentary) each day, and don't forget to keep to The Food Effect principles and rules laid out in Chapter 2 throughout the four weeks of this phase. As well as adhering to these rules, keep to the following few additional rules specific to the Attack Phase.

1. There should be no interchanging of meals between different categories (as explained above).

2. Make sure you have a glass of water with a tablespoon of apple cider vinegar soon after waking every day (stevia or xylitol can be added to sweeten the drink). This will kick-start your metabolism and digestive system ready for the day ahead.

3. The only fruits allowed during this phase are apples, oranges, pears, grapefruit and berries. Occasionally, a small portion of dried fruit (such as raisins) is specified. (Once you move on to the Lifestyle Phase, all fruits are allowed, apart from bananas.)

4. Keep to a maximum of two slices of wholemeal or rye or sourdough bread per day during this phase. Each day has already been designed this way for you; for example, if lunch is a sandwich, there won't be an option that includes a slice of toast for breakfast, so you don't have to think about this if you are following the specified meals. But if you choose to interchange meals, make sure you don't exceed two slices of bread across all meals per day.

5. The carbohydrates to stick to that are included in the 28-day plan are minimally processed unrefined carbs including oats, quinoa, sweet potato, brown rice, wholemeal bread, Ryvita crackers, brown rice cakes and oatcakes. There is no whole-wheat pasta or whole-grain breakfast cereal in this phase – these are introduced into the meal options for the Lifestyle Phase.

6. Salads can be dressed and seasoned with lemon juice, balsamic vinegar or apple cider vinegar, plus herbs, salt and pepper. No olive oil should be added to salads (unless specified in a given recipe), and definitely no rich sauces or creamy dressings.

7. Drink at least 2 litres of water a day.

8. You can have two coffees or teas with almond (or any plant-based milk with no added sugar) per day; all other hot drinks should be herbal teas.

9. You must have your mid-afternoon snack. Evening snacks are optional, however. Many of my clients find that they don't need them (or only have them on the odd night). You're certainly allowed it, but if you don't feel hungry after dinner on any given night, don't feel you must have it.

10. No mid-morning snacks – have a hot drink or herbal tea if you're peckish.

11. No cheat meals during the Attack Phase. (The Lifestyle Phase does, however, allow room for indulgences and being lenient on special occasions.)

12. Weigh yourself every morning (without clothes on) during these 28 days. As explained in the general rules, once you move on to the Lifestyle Phase, you'll only be expected to weigh yourself once a week.

The benefits of weighing yourself

A study in the *Journal of the Academy of Nutrition and Dietetics* found that weighing yourself every day leads to greater adoption of weight-control behaviours, and produces greater weight loss compared with weighing yourself most days of the week. The study showed that the more frequently people weighed themselves, the more 'cognitive restraint' they had for consuming unhealthy, fatty foods. In other words, you'll be less likely to grab a handful of greasy chips or a bag of crisps at work if you know it's going to make the scales go in the wrong direction. This is especially helpful to get you going in the first four weeks of The Food Effect Diet Vegan, which are the strictest, and occur when you're just beginning to cut out all the bad stuff and change your eating habits for good.

You need as much discipline during this time as possible, and knowing that you have to step on the scales every morning definitely helps. Another added benefit of this is that it gives real encouragement to keep going as you see the number on the scales going down.

That being said, however, it's unrealistic to expect to see a drop every single day, so don't get despondent or expect this to happen – your weight might stay the same for several days, then you'll see a sudden drop. Also, things like salt intake or, for women, having periods, can cause the body to retain more fluid and thus nudge up the number on the scales for a day or two. Don't worry, as long as you stick to your plan and keep going, you'll see the overall number drop by the end of the four weeks.

Once you've finished the Attack Phase, I recommend that you weigh yourself once a week when you've moved on to The Food Effect Diet Vegan Lifestyle Phase. Weekly monitoring will allow you to catch small weight gains, and initiate corrective behavioural and dietary changes, without obsessing about your weight.

Despite these additional rules, once you get started you'll be surprised at how doable it all is.

The Attack Phase plan

Day 1

Breakfast
Chocolate Chia Seed Pudding (page 215)
Serve with 75g strawberries or blueberries
Coffee or tea with almond milk, or herbal tea

Mid-morning
Tea, coffee or herbal tea – you can add almond or any other
plant-based milk (unsweetened)

Lunch
Chickpea Salad: combine 1 small tin or ½ large tin chickpeas
(120g drained weight), 1 red pepper, deseeded and diced, or 2
chopped tomatoes and unlimited mixed salad leaves, drizzle
with balsamic vinegar or lemon juice, plus herbs, salt and
black pepper.
Serve with 3 Ryvita crackers or brown rice cakes

Afternoon snack
1 apple or pear, plus 12 almonds
Mug of herbal tea

Dinner
Quinoa Salad with Roasted Vegetables (page 225) – save half
for tomorrow's lunch
Serve with a mixed green salad drizzled with balsamic vinegar

Evening snack
30g dark chocolate (70 per cent cocoa or above) plus fresh fruit
(1 apple, or pear or orange)
Mug of herbal tea

Day 2

Breakfast
150g soya natural yoghurt (unsweetened)
75g mixed berries (blueberries, blackberries, strawberries)
Drizzle of agave syrup (1–2 tsp)
Coffee or tea with almond milk, or herbal tea

Mid-morning
Tea, coffee or herbal tea

Lunch
Quinoa Salad with Roasted Vegetables (left over from last
night's supper)
1 large apple

Afternoon snack
2 celery sticks topped with 1 flat tbsp peanut or almond
butter (15g)
Mug of herbal tea

Dinner
Vegan Chinese 'Chicken' Stir-Fry (page 235)
Serve with 125g cooked brown rice
Mixed green salad drizzled with balsamic vinegar

Evening snack
Fresh fruit (apple or pear or orange) plus 12 almonds or
cashew nuts
Mug of herbal tea

Day 3

Breakfast
Dairy-Free Protein Parfait (page 218)
Coffee or tea with almond milk, or herbal tea

Mid-morning
Tea, coffee or herbal tea

Lunch
Wild Rice and Avocado Salad: combine unlimited salad leaves, a large chunk of chopped cucumber, 2 spring onions, 1 grated or chopped raw carrot, ½ sliced avocado, fresh coriander and 125g cooked wild or brown rice. Season with salt and pepper. Dress with lemon juice or balsamic vinegar.

Afternoon snack
Pre-cut carrot sticks, plus 2 tbsp reduced-fat hummus or The Food Effect Spinach Hummus (page 252)
Mug of herbal tea

Dinner
Spicy Stuffed Sweet Potato (page 229)
Serve with mixed green salad or fresh spinach leaves, drizzled with balsamic vinegar

Evening snack
Baked apple with pecan nuts: 1 baked apple (or fresh if preferred), sprinkled with stevia or xylitol and cinnamon, plus 2 tbsp chopped pecan nuts.
Mug of herbal tea

Day 4

Breakfast
Avocado Toast (page 217)
Serve with sliced tomato, seasoned with salt and pepper
Coffee or tea with almond milk, or herbal tea

Mid-morning
Tea, coffee or herbal tea

Lunch
Falafel and Sweetcorn Salad: 3 shop-bought baked falafel
balls (for example GOSH falafel), cut into halves, 1 small tin
sweetcorn (150g), mixed salad/vegetables (chopped lettuce/
spinach leaves, cucumber, cherry tomatoes, grated carrot, red
or yellow pepper), tossed with balsamic vinegar or lemon juice.
Season with salt, pepper and chilli powder (optional).

Afternoon snack
1 apple or pear, plus 12 raw almonds or cashew nuts
Mug of herbal tea

Dinner
Protein-Packed Green Skinny Noodle Bowl (page 232)

Evening snack
150g natural soya yoghurt (unsweetened) plus 75g blueberries,
add stevia and cinnamon
Mug of herbal tea

Day 5

Breakfast
1 slice wholemeal toast or sourdough bread
2 tbsp Blueberry Chia Seed Jam (page 217)
Coffee or tea with almond milk, or herbal tea

Mid-morning
Tea, coffee or herbal tea

Lunch
Avocado, Spinach and Strawberry Salad with Sweet Poppy Seed
Dressing (page 231)

Afternoon snack
2 brown rice cakes or vegan oatcakes plus 2 tbsp (30g) reduced-
fat hummus
Mug of herbal tea

Dinner
Vegan Stuffed Pepper (page 234)
Serve with 125g cooked brown rice and mixed green salad
drizzled with balsamic vinegar

Evening snack
25g mixed dried fruit and nuts
Mug of herbal tea

Day 6

Breakfast
Perfect Porridge (page 216)
Serve with 1 tbsp mixed seeds (sunflower, pumpkin, flaxseeds)
Coffee or tea with almond milk, or herbal tea

Mid-morning
Tea, coffee or herbal tea

Lunch
Mixed Bean Salad: combine 1 small tin (150g) or ½ × 400g
tin mixed bean salad, 1 red pepper, deseeded and diced or 2
chopped tomatoes and unlimited mixed salad leaves.
Drizzle with balsamic/apple cider vinegar plus herbs, salt and
black pepper. Serve with 3 Ryvita crackers or brown rice cakes

Afternoon snack
1 orange plus 12 raw cashew nuts
Mug of herbal tea

Dinner
Teriyaki Tofu (page 216)
Serve with unlimited mixed stir-fried or roasted vegetables
(cooked with minimal oil/spray oil)

Evening snack
30g dark chocolate (70 per cent cocoa or above) plus 75g
strawberries
Mug of herbal tea

Day 7

Breakfast
Egg-Free Coconut French Toast (page 215)
Serve with 75g sliced strawberries
Coffee or tea with almond milk, or herbal tea

Mid-morning
Tea, coffee or herbal tea

Lunch
Quinoa Chickpea Salad: 185g cooked quinoa, 1 small tin or
½ large tin chickpeas (120g drained weight), mixed salad
(diced cucumber, tomato and red pepper) and 1 tbsp vegan
mayonnaise, mixed with lemon juice, salt and pepper

Afternoon snack
30g low-fat (salted) popcorn (for example Propercorn)
Mug of herbal tea

Dinner
Vegan Cauliflower Cheese (page 233)
Serve with mixed green salad drizzled with balsamic vinegar

Evening snack
Baked apple with pecan nuts: 1 baked apple (or fresh if
preferred), sprinkled with stevia or xylitol and cinnamon, plus
2 tbsp chopped pecan nuts
Mug of herbal tea

Day 8

Breakfast
150g soya natural yoghurt (unsweetened)
75g mixed berries (blueberries, blackberries and strawberries)
Drizzle of agave syrup (1–2 tsp)
Coffee or tea with almond milk, or herbal tea

Mid-morning
Tea, coffee or herbal tea

Lunch
Hummus Salad Sandwich: 2 slices wholemeal bread filled with
salad (fresh spinach leaves) and sliced tomato, season with salt
and pepper, 2 tbsp reduced-fat hummus and pre-cut carrot
sticks on the side

Afternoon snack
1 apple, plus 12 almonds
Mug of herbal tea

Dinner
Avocado, Spinach and Strawberry Salad with Sweet Poppy Seed
Dressing (page 231)
Serve with 1 vegan burger (for example: Beyond Meat Burger
or Fry's vegan burger)

Evening snack
30g dark chocolate (70 per cent cocoa or above) plus fresh fruit
(1 apple, or pear or orange)
Mug of herbal tea

Day 9

Breakfast
Chocolate Chia Seed Pudding (page 215)
Serve with 75g strawberries or blueberries
Coffee or tea with almond milk, or herbal tea

Mid-morning
Tea, coffee or herbal tea

Lunch
Roasted Vegetable, Chickpea and Sunflower Seed Salad
(page 226)

Afternoon snack
1 orange, plus 12 raw cashew nuts or almonds
Mug of herbal tea

Dinner
Chinese-Style Tofu and Kale (page 236)
Serve with 125g cooked brown rice

Evening snack
2 vegan oatcakes, plus 2 tbsp (30g) reduced-fat hummus or The
Food Effect Spinach Hummus (page 252)
Mug of herbal tea

Day 10

Breakfast
Perfect Porridge (page 216)
Serve with 1 mini-box (14g) or 2 tbsp raisins
Coffee or tea with almond milk, or herbal tea

Mid-morning
Tea, coffee or herbal tea

Lunch
Quinoa, Falafel and Avocado Salad: 185g cooked quinoa, 3
shop-bought baked falafel balls (for example GOSH brand),
diced cucumber, tomato, red pepper and ¼ avocado, top with
lemon juice, salt and pepper

Afternoon snack
1 pear, plus 2 vegan oatcakes
Mug of herbal tea

Dinner
Spicy Stuffed Sweet Potato (page 229)
Serve with a mixed green salad or fresh spinach leaves, drizzled
with balsamic vinegar

Evening snack
Fresh fruit (1 apple, pear or orange), plus 12 almonds
Mug of herbal tea

Day 11

Breakfast
Avocado Toast (page 217)
Serve with sliced tomato, seasoned with salt and pepper
Coffee or tea with almond milk, or herbal tea

Mid-morning
Tea, coffee or herbal tea

Lunch
Mixed Bean Salad: combine 1 small tin (150g) or ½ × 400g tin
mixed bean salad, 1 red pepper, diced or 2 chopped tomatoes
and unlimited mixed salad leaves, drizzle with balsamic/apple
cider vinegar plus herbs, salt and black pepper
Serve with 1 apple or pear, or 3 Ryvita crackers

Afternoon snack
150g soya natural yoghurt (unsweetened), plus 75g blueberries
with stevia and cinnamon
Mug of herbal tea

Dinner
Green Bean and Butternut Casserole with Crunchy Peanut Butter
Sauce (page 238) – save the leftovers for tomorrow's lunch.
Serve with 125g cooked brown rice

Evening snack
Pear with Pecan Nuts: serve half a baked pear (or fresh if
preferred), sprinkled with stevia and cinnamon, and 2 tbsp
crushed pecan nuts
Mug of herbal tea

Day 12

Breakfast
Apple Pie Overnight Oats (page 214)
Coffee or tea with almond milk, or herbal tea

Mid-morning
Tea, coffee or herbal tea

Lunch
Green Bean and Butternut Casserole with Crunchy Peanut
Butter Sauce (left over from last night's dinner)
Serve with mixed green salad, drizzled with balsamic vinegar

Afternoon snack
2 vegan oatcakes, plus 2 tbsp reduced-fat hummus (30g) or The
Food Effect Spinach Hummus (page 252)
Mug of herbal tea

Dinner
Teriyaki Tofu (page 234)
Serve with unlimited mixed stir-fried or roasted vegetables
(cooked with minimal oil/spray oil)

Evening snack
25g mixed dried fruit and nuts
Mug of herbal tea

Day 13

Breakfast
1 slice wholemeal or sourdough bread, toasted
2 tbsp Blueberry Chia Seed Jam (page 217)
Coffee or tea with almond milk, or herbal tea

Mid-morning
Tea, coffee or herbal tea

Lunch
Falafel and Sweetcorn Salad: 3 shop-bought baked falafel
balls (for example GOSH brand), cut into halves, 1 small tin
sweetcorn (150g), mixed salad/vegetables (chopped lettuce/
spinach leaves, cucumber, cherry tomatoes, grated carrot, red/
yellow pepper), tossed with balsamic vinegar or lemon juice.
Season with salt, pepper and chilli powder (optional)

Afternoon snack
2 celery sticks, topped with 1 level tbsp peanut or almond
butter (15g)
Mug of herbal tea

Dinner
Quinoa Salad with Roasted Vegetables (page 225) – save half
for tomorrow's lunch
Serve with mixed green salad drizzled with balsamic vinegar

Evening snack
30g dark chocolate (70 per cent cocoa or above), plus 75g
strawberries or mixed berries
Mug of herbal tea

Day 14

Breakfast
Egg-Free Coconut French Toast (page 215)
Serve with 75g sliced strawberries
Coffee or tea with almond milk, or herbal tea

Mid-morning
Tea, coffee or herbal tea

Lunch
Quinoa Salad with Roasted Vegetables (left over from last
night's dinner)
1 large apple

Afternoon snack
30g low-fat (salted) popcorn (for example Propercorn)
Mug of herbal tea

Dinner
Spicy Stuffed Sweet Potato (page 229)
Mixed green salad, drizzled with balsamic vinegar

Evening snack
Strawberries with Pecan Nuts: 75g sliced strawberries, plus 2
tbsp crushed pecan nuts, sprinkled with stevia or xylitol
Mug of herbal tea

Day 15

Breakfast
1 slice wholemeal or sourdough bread, toasted

1 tbsp vegan cream cheese (almond milk/cashew nut-based –
for example Nush brand)

1 apple or orange, or ½ grapefruit – top with stevia or xylitol
(optional)

Coffee or tea with almond milk, or herbal tea

Mid-morning
Tea, coffee or herbal tea

Lunch
Avocado and Chickpea Salad (page 225)

Afternoon snack
30g low-fat (salted) popcorn (for example Propercorn)

Mug of herbal tea

Dinner
1 vegan burger (for example Beyond Meat Burger or Fry's
vegan burger)

Fresh spinach/salad leaves, drizzled with balsamic vinegar

Diced fresh tomatoes, cucumber or red pepper, seasoned with
salt and pepper

125g cooked quinoa or brown rice

Evening snack
30g dark chocolate (70 per cent cocoa or above), plus fruit
(1 apple, or pear or orange)

Mug of herbal tea

Day 16

Breakfast
Apple Pie Overnight Oats (page 214)
Coffee or tea with almond milk, or herbal tea

Mid-morning
Tea, coffee or herbal tea

Lunch
Quinoa, Falafel and Avocado Salad: 185g cooked quinoa, 3 shop-bought baked falafel balls (for example GOSH brand), diced cucumber, tomato, red pepper and ¼ avocado. Top with lemon juice, salt and pepper

Afternoon snack
1 apple, plus 2 Ryvita or vegan oatcakes
Mug of herbal tea

Dinner
Tofu, Spinach and Strawberry Salad with Sweet Poppy Seed Dressing (page 230)

Evening snack
25g mixed dried fruit and nuts
Mug of herbal tea

Day 17

Breakfast
1 slice wholemeal or sourdough bread, toasted
2 tbsp Blueberry Chia Seed Jam (page 217)
Coffee or tea with almond milk, or herbal tea

Mid-morning
Tea, coffee or herbal tea

Lunch
Roasted Vegetable, Chickpea and Sunflower Seed Salad
(page 226)

Afternoon snack
1 apple or orange, plus 12 almonds
Mug of herbal tea

Dinner
Vegan Chinese 'Chicken' Stir-Fry (page 235)
Serve with 125g cooked brown rice
Mixed green salad drizzled with balsamic vinegar

Evening snack
Pear with Pecan Nuts: serve ½ baked pear (or fresh if
preferred), sprinkled with stevia and cinnamon, and 2 tbsp
crushed pecan nuts
Mug of herbal tea

Day 18

Breakfast
Chocolate Chia Seed Pudding (page 215)
Coffee or tea with almond milk, or herbal tea

Mid-morning
Tea, coffee or herbal tea

Lunch
Avocado and Almond Salad (page 237)

Afternoon snack
1 pear, plus 12 cashew nuts
Mug of herbal tea

Dinner
Chinese-Style Tofu and Kale (page 236)
Serve with 125g cooked brown rice

Evening snack
150g natural soya yoghurt (unsweetened) plus 75g blueberries,
add stevia and cinnamon
Mug of herbal tea

Day 19

Breakfast
150g soya natural yoghurt (unsweetened)
75g mixed berries (blueberries, blackberries, strawberries)
Drizzle of agave syrup (1–2 tsp)
Coffee or tea with almond milk, or herbal tea

Mid-morning
Tea, coffee or herbal tea

Lunch
Avocado and Chickpea Salad (page 225)

Afternoon snack:
2 dried figs, plus 12 almonds
Mug of herbal tea

Dinner
1 serving Slow-Cooker Sweet Potato Vegan Chilli (page 237) –
pack leftovers for tomorrow's lunch and/or freeze any extra
Serve on a large bowl of fresh spinach leaves or steamed green
beans, drizzled with balsamic vinegar or low-sodium soy sauce

Evening snack
Baked Apple with Pecan Nuts: 1 baked apple (or fresh if
preferred), sprinkled with stevia, cinnamon and 2 tbsp chopped
pecan nuts
Mug of herbal tea

Day 20

Breakfast
Avocado Toast (page 217)
Serve with sliced tomato, seasoned with salt and pepper
Coffee or tea with almond milk, or herbal tea

Mid-morning
Tea, coffee or herbal tea

Lunch
1 serving Slow-Cooker Sweet Potato Vegan Chilli (left over
from yesterday's supper)
Serve with mixed green salad drizzled with balsamic vinegar or
low-sodium soy sauce

Afternoon snack
150g soya natural yoghurt (unsweetened), plus 75g blueberries
with stevia and cinnamon
Mug of herbal tea

Dinner
2 Beetroot Burgers (page 227) or 2 Cauliflower and Chickpea
Burgers (page 228) – make full recipe and save leftovers for
Day 22 lunch
Serve with fresh spinach leaves drizzled with balsamic vinegar
and Miraculous Butternut Squash Mash (page 252)

Evening snack
Fresh fruit (1 apple, or pear or orange), plus 12 almonds
Mug of herbal tea

Day 21

Breakfast
1 slice wholemeal or sourdough bread, toasted, or 3 Ryvita

2 tbsp vegan cream cheese (almond milk/cashew nut-based –
for example Nush brand)

Sliced tomato or cucumber, seasoned with salt and pepper

Coffee or tea with almond milk, or herbal tea

Mid-morning
Tea, coffee or herbal tea

Lunch
Mixed Bean Salad: combine 1 small tin (150g) or ½ × 400g
tin mixed bean salad, 1 red pepper, deseeded and diced, and
unlimited mixed salad leaves. Drizzle with balsamic vinegar,
plus herbs, salt and black pepper

1 apple or pear

Afternoon snack
2 vegan oatcakes, plus 2 tbsp reduced-fat hummus or The Food
Effect Spinach Hummus (page 252)

Mug of herbal tea

Dinner
Vegan Stuffed Pepper (page 234)

Serve with 125g cooked brown rice and a mixed green salad
drizzled with balsamic vinegar

Evening snack
30g dark chocolate (70 per cent cocoa or above), plus 1 orange

Mug of herbal tea

Day 22

Breakfast
Perfect Porridge (page 216)
Serve with 1 tbsp mixed seeds (sunflower, pumpkin, flaxseeds)
Coffee or tea with almond milk, or herbal tea

Mid-morning
Tea, coffee or herbal tea

Lunch
2 Beetroot Burgers or 2 Cauliflower and Chickpea Burgers –
left over from Day 20
Serve with fresh spinach leaves and chopped cucumber
(unlimited), drizzled with balsamic vinegar or lemon juice plus
salt and pepper. Ketchup (reduced sugar) on the side (optional)

Afternoon snack
1 apple, plus 12 almonds
Mug of herbal tea

Dinner
Quinoa Salad with Roasted Vegetables (page 225) – save half
for tomorrow's lunch
Serve with mixed green salad, drizzled with balsamic vinegar

Evening snack
150g natural soya yoghurt (unsweetened) plus 75g strawberries,
add stevia and cinnamon
Mug of herbal tea

Day 23

Breakfast
Apple Pie Overnight Oats (page 214)
Coffee or tea with almond milk, or herbal tea

Mid-morning
Tea, coffee or herbal tea

Lunch
Quinoa Salad with Roasted Vegetables – left over from last
night's dinner
1 large apple

Afternoon snack
Pre-cut carrot sticks, plus 2 tbsp reduced-fat hummus or The
Food Effect Spinach Hummus (page 252)
Mug of herbal tea

Dinner
Protein-Packed Super-Green Skinny Noodle Bowl (page 232)

Evening snack
25g mixed dried fruit and nuts
Mug of herbal tea

Day 24

Breakfast

1 slice wholemeal or sourdough bread, toasted or 3 Ryvita

2 tbsp vegan cream cheese (almond milk/cashew nut-based –
for example Nush brand) mixed with stevia and cinnamon
(optional)

150g mixed berries

Coffee or tea with almond milk, or herbal tea

Mid-morning

Tea, coffee or herbal tea

Lunch

Avocado, Spinach and Strawberry Salad with Sweet Poppy Seed
Dressing (page 231)

Afternoon snack

30g low-fat (salted) popcorn (for example Propercorn)

Mug of herbal tea

Dinner

Vegan Cauliflower Cheese (page 233)

Serve with fresh salad leaves, drizzled with balsamic vinegar
(unlimited)

Evening snack

30g dark chocolate (70 per cent cocoa or above), plus fruit
(1 apple, or pear or orange)

Mug of herbal tea

Day 25

Breakfast
Avocado Toast (page 217)
Serve with sliced tomato, seasoned with salt and pepper
Coffee or tea with almond milk, or herbal tea

Mid-morning
Tea, coffee or herbal tea

Lunch
Falafel and Sweetcorn Salad: 3 shop-bought baked falafel
balls (for example GOSH brand), cut into halves, 1 small tin
sweetcorn (150g), mixed salad/vegetables (chopped lettuce/
spinach leaves, cucumber, cherry tomatoes, grated carrot, red/
yellow pepper), drizzled with balsamic vinegar or lemon juice.
Season with salt, pepper and chilli powder (optional)

Afternoon snack
150g soya natural yoghurt, plus 75g strawberries mixed with
stevia and cinnamon
Mug of herbal tea

Dinner
Vegan Chinese 'Chicken' Stir-Fry (page 235)
Serve with 125g cooked brown rice
Mixed green salad drizzled with balsamic vinegar

Evening snack
Baked Apple with Pecan Nuts: 1 baked apple (or fresh if
preferred) sprinkled with stevia and cinnamon, and 2 tbsp
chopped pecan nuts
Mug of herbal tea

Day 26

Breakfast
Perfect Porridge (page 216)
Serve with 75g fresh blueberries
Coffee or tea with almond milk, or herbal tea

Mid-morning
Tea, coffee or herbal tea

Lunch
Avocado and Almond Salad (page 237)

Afternoon snack
Pre-cut carrot sticks, plus 2 tbsp reduced-fat hummus or The
Food Effect Spinach Hummus (page 252)
Mug of herbal tea

Dinner
2 Beetroot Burgers (page 227) or 2 Cauliflower and Chickpea
Burgers (page 228) – save leftovers for tomorrow's lunch
Serve with fresh spinach leaves drizzled with balsamic vinegar
and Butternut Squash Miraculous Mash (page 252)

Evening snack
30g dark chocolate (70 per cent cocoa or above), plus
1 apple or pear
Mug of herbal tea

Day 27

Breakfast
Chocolate Chia Seed Pudding (page 215)
Coffee or tea with almond milk, or herbal tea

Mid-morning
Tea, coffee or herbal tea

Lunch
2 Beetroot Burgers or 2 Cauliflower and Chickpea Burgers –
left over from yesterday's dinner

Serve with fresh spinach leaves and chopped cucumber
(unlimited), drizzled with balsamic vinegar or lemon juice plus
salt and pepper. Ketchup (reduced sugar) on the side (optional)

Afternoon snack
2 vegan oatcakes, plus 2 tbsp reduced-fat hummus or The Food
Effect Spinach Hummus (page 252).
Mug of herbal tea

Dinner
Teriyaki Tofu (page 234)
Serve with unlimited mixed stir-fried or roasted vegetables
(cooked with minimal oil/spray oil)

Evening snack
Fresh fruit (1 apple, or pear or orange), plus 12 almonds
Mug of herbal tea

Day 28

Breakfast
Egg-Free Coconut French Toast (page 215)
Serve with 75g sliced strawberries
Coffee or tea with almond milk, or herbal tea

Mid-morning
Tea, coffee or herbal tea

Lunch
Mixed Bean Salad: combine 1 small (150g) or ½ × 400g tin
mixed bean salad, 1 red pepper deseeded and chopped, or 2
chopped tomatoes and unlimited mixed salad leaves. Drizzle
with balsamic vinegar, and season with herbs, salt and
black pepper
Serve with 3 Ryvita crackers or brown rice cakes

Afternoon snack
1 apple, plus 12 almonds
Mug of herbal tea

Dinner
Chinese-Style Tofu and Kale (page 236)
Serve with 125g cooked brown rice

Evening snack
30g dark chocolate (70 per cent cocoa or above), plus
75g strawberries
Mug of herbal tea

CHAPTER 12

Phase 2, Continued Weight Loss and Maintenance

The Food Effect Diet Vegan Lifestyle and meal options

After four weeks on Phase 1, the Attack Phase, you'll switch to the more liberal version of the diet and start living The Food Effect Diet Vegan Lifestyle. You'll reintroduce even more healthy carbs, including whole-wheat pasta and low-sugar, whole-grain breakfast cereals. The weight loss will slow slightly from Phase 1, but should still be around 1–2lb per week until you reach your goal weight. At this point, this way of eating will have become a way of life for you – your regular healthy lifestyle, rather than a weight-loss programme. You'll be knowledgeable enough about how The Food Effect Diet Vegan works to enjoy all the flexibility of the plan, while staying slim and enjoying your food.

How to follow the Lifestyle Phase

To follow The Food Effect Diet Vegan Lifestyle, simply choose any one breakfast, lunch, mid-afternoon snack, supper and evening snack per day to make up your day's worth of eating. Obviously, you can eat less than this (for example, if you don't feel you need or want an evening snack after dinner every day, or if you want fewer crackers than specified with lunch), but you cannot have more than this per day. This way, you'll never exceed the calorie cap to make you gain weight or prevent you from losing it.

Unlike during the Attack Phase, you're now allowed more than two pieces of any wholemeal/rye/sourdough bread per day (as long as it fits into the meal options). So, for example, you can choose a breakfast option that includes a piece of toast, and lunch might be a sandwich. This doesn't mean that you should aim to do this every day, as variety is always good, but you are certainly allowed to do so, and it won't compromise your weight as long as you keep to the portions specified in the options.

There may be times once you're on the Lifestyle Phase, during your continued weight loss (or maintenance) regime, when you'll 'fall off the wagon'. This is entirely normal – we're all human. You might over-indulge during a festive season or while on holiday. Stressful times can also trigger many people to overeat (which again is completely normal and human), and as a result gain some weight. When these situations arise, I suggest that you switch back to the Attack Phase, even if it's just for a few days or a week – however long you need until you lose the weight you gained, and get yourself back on track. That's how I designed The Food Effect Diet – the two phases allow enough flexibility to acknowledge and accommodate real life.

For ease, while all the options that follow are for The Food Effect Diet Vegan Lifestyle Phase, I've also included those that are suitable for the Attack Phase, so that if you wish to choose stricter options for certain meals (for example, if you've got a big dinner in the evening and want a lighter breakfast or lunch), you can simply choose an option that is Attack Phase friendly. That way you'll stay on track easily, throughout your new way of life.

The Lifestyle Phase plan

Attack Phase recipes are indicated by an asterisk (*).

BREAKFAST

* Chocolate Chia Seed Pudding (page 215)
Serve with 75g fresh strawberries or blueberries
Coffee or tea with almond milk, or herbal tea

* Dairy-Free Protein Parfait (page 218)
Coffee or tea with almond milk, or herbal tea

* Avocado Toast (page 217)
Serve with sliced tomatoes, seasoned with salt and black pepper
Coffee or tea with almond milk, or herbal tea

* 1 slice wholemeal or sourdough bread, toasted
2 tbsp Blueberry Chia Seed Jam (page 217)
Coffee or tea with almond milk, or herbal tea

* 150g soya natural yoghurt (unsweetened)
75g mixed berries (blueberries, blackberries, strawberries)
Drizzle of agave syrup (1–2 tsp)
Coffee or tea with almond milk, or herbal tea

* 1 slice wholemeal or sourdough bread, toasted
1 tbsp vegan cream cheese (almond milk/cashew nut-based – for example Nush brand)
1 apple or orange, or ½ grapefruit – top with stevia or xylitol (optional)
Coffee or tea with almond milk, or herbal tea

* Perfect Porridge (page 216)
Serve with 1 tbsp mixed seeds (sunflower, pumpkin, flaxseeds)
Coffee or tea with almond milk, or herbal tea

* Egg-Free Coconut French Toast (page 215)
Serve with 75g sliced strawberries
Coffee or tea with almond milk, or herbal tea

* Perfect Porridge (page 216)
Serve with 1 mini-box (14g) or 2 tbsp raisins
Coffee or tea with almond milk, or herbal tea

* Apple Pie Overnight Oats (page 214)
Coffee or tea with almond milk, or herbal tea

* Perfect Porridge (page 216)
Serve with 75g blueberries
Coffee or tea with almond milk, or herbal tea

* 1 slice wholemeal bread, toasted or 3 Ryvita crackers
2 tbsp vegan cream cheese (almond milk/cashew nut-based – for example Nush brand)
Sliced fresh tomato, seasoned with herbs, salt and pepper
Coffee or tea with almond milk, or herbal tea

* 1 slice wholemeal bread, toasted, or 3 Ryvita crackers
2 tbsp vegan cream cheese (almond milk/cashew nut-based – for example Nush brand)
150g mixed berries
Coffee or tea with almond milk, or herbal tea

Porridge cooked in microwave using 1 packet instant oats (no added sugar), or 50g uncooked oats, plus 180ml almond milk, stevia or xylitol and a pinch of salt (allow to stand for a few minutes before eating – it swells). Once cooked, add 1 level tbsp peanut or almond butter, stevia and cinnamon
Coffee or tea with almond milk, or herbal tea

2 Weetabix, topped with stevia and cinnamon
240ml unsweetened almond milk
1 mini-box (14g) or 2 tbsp raisins
Coffee or tea with almond milk, or herbal tea

150g soya natural yoghurt (unsweetened)
Serve with 75g mixed berries, plus 1 tbsp pumpkin or sunflower seeds
Drizzle of agave syrup (1 tsp) with cinnamon
Coffee or tea with almond milk, or herbal tea

40g whole-grain cereal (such as Kellogg's All-Bran Original or
Bran Flakes)
240ml unsweetened almond milk
75g fresh blueberries
Coffee or tea with almond milk, or herbal tea

125g soya natural yoghurt (unsweetened) – add stevia and cinnamon
25g Kellogg's All-Bran Original or Bran Flakes
75g blueberries or 1 mini-box (14g) or 2 tbsp raisins
Coffee or tea with almond milk, or herbal tea

Almond Mango Yoghurt: 150g soya natural yoghurt (unsweetened),
topped with 75g chopped fresh mango and 1 tbsp toasted flaked
almonds. Drizzle of agave syrup (1–2 tsp), plus a sprinkling of
ginger/cinnamon
Coffee or tea with almond milk, or herbal tea

150g soya natural yoghurt (unsweetened) – add stevia or xylitol
150g fruit (such as cut-up melon, pineapple, strawberries or
other berries)
3 Ryvita crackers or 1 slice wholemeal bread, toasted
Coffee or tea with almond milk, or herbal tea

1 slice wholemeal or sourdough bread, toasted or 3 Ryvita crackers
1 tbsp vegan cream cheese (almond milk/cashew nut-based) mixed
with stevia and cinnamon
150g diced pineapple (or any fruit, such as strawberries and melon)
Coffee or tea with almond milk, or herbal tea

½ wholemeal bagel or 1 slice wholemeal bread, toasted
1 level tbsp peanut or almond butter
1 apple
Coffee or tea with almond milk, or herbal tea

Nutty Vanilla Overnight Oats (page 219)
Coffee or tea with almond milk, or herbal tea

1 Healthy Wholesome Energy Bar (page 220)
Coffee or tea with almond milk, or herbal tea

1 Guilt-Free Courgette Muffin (page 221)
Coffee or tea with almond milk, or herbal tea

Blueberry Bliss Protein Shake (page 218)

The Food Effect Green Power Shake (page 222)

The Food Effect Chocolate Peanut Butter Power Shake (page 222)

The Food Effect Chocolate Green Power Shake (page 223)

Sweet Potato Pie Smoothie (page 224)

MID-MORNING

Tea, coffee or herbal tea – you can add almond or any other plant-
based milk (unsweetened).

LUNCH

* Chickpea Salad: combine 1 small tin or ½ large tin chickpeas (120g drained weight), 1 red pepper, diced or 2 chopped tomatoes and unlimited mixed salad leaves
Drizzle with balsamic vinegar or lemon juice, plus herbs, salt and black pepper
Serve with 3 Ryvita crackers or brown rice cakes

* Quinoa Salad with Roasted Vegetables (page 225)
1 large apple

* Wild Rice and Avocado Salad: combine unlimited salad leaves, a large chunk of chopped cucumber, 1–2 spring onions, 1 grated or chopped raw carrot, ½ sliced avocado, fresh coriander and 125g cooked wild or brown rice. Season with salt and pepper. Dress with lemon juice or balsamic vinegar

* Avocado, Spinach and Strawberry Salad with Sweet Poppy Seed Dressing (page 231)

* Mixed Bean Salad: combine 1 small tin (150g) or ½ x 400g tin mixed bean salad, 1 red pepper, diced, or 2 chopped tomatoes and unlimited mixed salad leaves. Drizzle with balsamic/apple cider vinegar plus herbs, salt and black pepper
Serve with 1 apple or pear, or 3 Ryvita crackers or brown rice cakes

* Quinoa Chickpea Salad: 185g cooked quinoa, 1 small tin or ½ x 400g tin chickpeas.
Mixed salad (diced cucumber, tomato and red pepper). Dress with 1 tbsp vegan mayonnaise, mixed with lemon juice, salt and pepper

* Hummus Salad Sandwich: 2 slices of wholemeal bread filled with salad (fresh spinach leaves and sliced tomato), 2 tbsp reduced-fat

hummus, and season with salt and pepper
Pre-cut carrot sticks on the side

* Roasted Vegetable, Chickpea and Sunflower Seed Salad (page 226)

* Quinoa, Falafel and Avocado Salad: 185g cooked quinoa, 3 shop-bought healthy baked falafel balls (for example GOSH brand), diced cucumber, tomato, red pepper and ¼ avocado. Top with lemon juice, salt and pepper

* Green Bean and Butternut Casserole with Crunchy Peanut Butter Sauce (page 238)
Serve with mixed green salad, drizzled with balsamic vinegar

* Falafel and Sweetcorn Salad: 3 shop-bought baked falafel (for example GOSH brand), cut into halves, 1 small tin sweetcorn (150g), mixed salad/vegetables (chopped lettuce/spinach leaves, cucumber, cherry tomatoes, grated carrot, red/yellow pepper), drizzled with balsamic vinegar or lemon juice. Season with salt, pepper and chilli powder (optional)

* Avocado and Chickpea Salad (page 225)

* Avocado and Almond Salad (page 237)

* 1 serving Slow-Cooker Sweet Potato Vegan Chilli (page 237)
Serve with a mixed green salad drizzled with balsamic vinegar

* 2 Beetroot Burgers (page 227) or 2 Cauliflower and Chickpea Burgers (page 228)
Serve with fresh spinach leaves and chopped cucumber (unlimited), drizzled with balsamic vinegar or lemon juice plus salt and pepper. Ketchup (reduced sugar) on the side (optional)

Couscous and Chickpea Salad: 125g cooked couscous, ½ × 400g tin chickpeas, mixed salad (diced cucumber, tomato, red peppers). Dressed with 1 tbsp tahini mixed with 1–2 tbsp lemon juice, plus salt and black pepper.

1 serving Quinoa, Wild Rice and Sweet Potato Salad (page 243)

The New Green Toast (page 244)
Serve with a mixed green salad drizzled with balsamic vinegar

2 Cauliflower and Chickpea Burgers (page 228) with Red Cabbage Slaw (page 262)
Mixed green salad, drizzled with balsamic vinegar

Cauliflower Burger Pitta (page 245)
Serve with a mixed green salad, drizzled with balsamic vinegar

1 serving Quinoa Salad with Avocado, Mango and Pomegranate (page 247)

1 serving Protein-Packed Pasta Dish (page 249)
Serve with fresh spinach leaves, unlimited

1 large bowl of soup (see recipes starting on page 253)
Serve with one small wholemeal roll and a green side salad

MID-AFTERNOON SNACKS

* 1 apple or pear, plus 12 almonds
Mug of herbal tea

* 1 apple, plus 2 Ryvita crackers or vegan oatcakes
Mug of herbal tea

* 2 celery sticks spread with 1 flat tbsp peanut or almond butter (15g)
Mug of herbal tea

* Pre-cut carrot sticks, plus 2 tbsp reduced-fat hummus or The Food
Effect Spinach Hummus (page 252)
Mug of herbal tea

* 2 brown rice cakes or vegan oatcakes plus 2 tbsp (30g) reduced-
fat hummus or The Food Effect Spinach Hummus (page 252)
Mug of herbal tea

* 1 orange, plus 12 raw almonds or cashew nuts
Mug of herbal tea

* 1 pear, plus 2 vegan oatcakes
Mug of herbal tea

* 150g soya natural yoghurt (unsweetened), plus 75g blueberries
mixed with stevia and cinnamon
Mug of herbal tea

* 150g soya natural yoghurt, plus 75g strawberries mixed with
stevia and cinnamon
Mug of herbal tea

* 2 dried figs, plus 12 almonds
Mug of herbal tea

* 30g low-fat (salted) popcorn (for example Propercorn)
Mug of herbal tea

2 tangerines plus 12 raw cashew nuts
Mug of herbal tea

Small bunch red grapes (50g), plus 12 almonds or 30 pistachio nuts
Mug of herbal tea

2 vegan oatcakes, plus 1 level tbsp peanut or almond butter
Mug of herbal tea

1 mini-box (14g) or 2 tbsp raisins, plus 12 almonds or cashew nuts
Mug of herbal tea

2 plums, plus 12 almonds or cashew nuts
Mug of herbal tea

5 dried apricots or prunes, plus 12 almonds
Mug of herbal tea

3 prunes or dried apricots, plus 6 walnuts
Mug of herbal tea

2 tangerines or plums, plus 1 tbsp pumpkin seeds
Mug of herbal tea

1 Nākd bar plus 1 small apple
Mug of herbal tea

Carrot, celery, cucumber and red pepper crudités, plus 2 tbsp
reduced-fat hummus
Mug of herbal tea

2 brown rice cakes, Ryvita crackers or Corn Thins, plus ½ avocado
Mug of herbal tea

2 vegan oatcakes, plus 1 level tbsp peanut or almond butter (15g)
Mug of herbal tea

2 vegan oatcakes each topped with 1 tbsp guacamole (page 241)
Mug of herbal tea

1 medium almond milk latte
1 large apple or pear

Blueberry Bliss Protein Shake (page 218)

¼ cup Sweet-and-Spicy Crunchy Chickpeas (page 265)

1 Hummus-Stuffed Date (page 266), plus 1 apple

30g Sweet-and-Spicy Nuts (page 267)

1–2 Dairy-Free 'Ferrero Rocher' Balls (page 267)

1–2 Chocolate, Date and Tahini Truffles (page 269)

1 Guilt-Free Courgette Muffin (page 221)

1–2 All-Healthy Raw Chocolate Truffle Balls (page 269)

1–2 Raw Bakewell Tart Balls (page 270)

1 Chocolate Peanut Cluster (page 271), plus 1 serving fresh fruit

1 No-bake Fibre-Filled Brownie Bar (page 271)

1–2 Peanut Cookie Energy Balls (page 272)

1–2 Tropical Mango Energy Balls (page 273)

DINNERS

* Quinoa Salad with Roasted Vegetables (page 225)
Serve with a mixed green salad drizzled with balsamic vinegar

* Vegan Chinese 'Chicken' Stir-Fry (page 235)
Serve with 125g cooked brown rice
Mixed green salad drizzled with balsamic vinegar

* Spicy Stuffed Sweet Potato (page 229)
Serve with a mixed green salad, drizzled with balsamic vinegar or
low-sodium soy sauce

* Protein-Packed Green Skinny Noodle Bowl (page 232)

* Vegan Stuffed Pepper (page 234)
Serve with 125g cooked brown rice and a mixed green salad
drizzled with balsamic vinegar

* Teriyaki Tofu (page 234)
Serve with unlimited mixed stir-fried or roasted vegetables (cooked
with minimal oil/spray oil)

* Vegan Cauliflower Cheese (page 233)
Serve with a mixed green salad drizzled with balsamic vinegar

* Avocado, Spinach and Strawberry Salad with Sweet Poppy Seed
Dressing (page 231)
Serve with 1 vegan burger (for example Beyond Meat Burger or
Fry's vegan burger)

* Chinese-Style Tofu and Kale (page 236)
Serve with 125g cooked brown rice

* Green Bean and Butternut Casserole with Crunchy Peanut Butter Sauce (page 238)
Serve with 125g cooked brown rice

* 1 vegan burger (for example Beyond Meat Burger or Fry's vegan burger)
Fresh spinach/salad leaves, drizzled with balsamic vinegar
Diced fresh tomatoes, cucumber or red pepper, seasoned with salt and pepper
125g cooked quinoa or brown rice

* Tofu, Spinach and Strawberry Salad with Sweet Poppy Seed Dressing (page 230)

* 1 serving Slow-Cooker Sweet Potato Vegan Chilli (page 237)
Serve on a large bowl of fresh spinach leaves or steamed green beans

* 2 Beetroot Burgers (page 227) or 2 Cauliflower and Chickpea Burgers (page 228)
Serve with fresh spinach leaves drizzled with balsamic vinegar and Miraculous Butternut Squash Mash (page 252)

1 serving Pulled Barbecue Jackfruit (page 239) served with Red Cabbage Slaw (page 262)
125g cooked brown rice or white basmati rice
Serve with mixed green salad drizzled with balsamic vinegar

1 Barbecue Jackfruit Burger (page 240)
Serve with mixed salad leaves (unlimited), drizzled with balsamic vinegar

1 serving World-Famous Vegetable Tagine (page 241)
Serve with 125g cooked brown rice or white basmati rice or whole-wheat couscous

1 serving Super-Simple Spaghetti Dish (page 242)
Serve with a mixed green salad or on a bed of fresh spinach leaves
drizzled with balsamic vinegar or low-sodium soy sauce

1 serving Quinoa, Wild Rice and Sweet Potato Salad (page 243)

Cauliflower and Chickpea Burgers (page 228) served with Red
Cabbage Slaw (page 262)
Serve with 125g cooked brown rice or quinoa

Cauliflower Burger Pitta (page 245)
Serve with mixed salad leaves (unlimited), drizzled with
balsamic vinegar

1 serving Easiest Ever One-Pot Hummus Pasta (page 246)
Serve with a fresh salad or on a bed of fresh spinach leaves

1 serving Curried Root Vegetable and Lentil Casserole (page 246)
Serve with 125g cooked brown rice or white basmati rice or whole-
wheat couscous

1 serving Quinoa Salad with Avocado, Mango and Pomegranate
(page 247)

1 serving Healthy Hearty Minestrone (page 248)
Serve with pre-cut carrot or other vegetable sticks on the side
(unlimited)

1 serving Protein-Packed Pasta Dish (page 249)
Serve with fresh spinach leaves drizzled with balsamic vinegar

1 serving Vegetable Bolognaise (page 250)
Serve on a bed of spinach leaves drizzled with balsamic vinegar or
low-salt soy sauce

1 vegan burger (for example Fry's brand or Beyond Meat Burger)
Roasted vegetables such as courgettes, mushrooms, red peppers and
red onions, cooked with minimal oil or spray oil, and seasoned with
herbs, salt and pepper
1 small baked sweet potato (150g) or Miraculous Butternut Squash
Mash (page 252)

1 vegan burger (for example Fry's brand or Beyond Meat Burger)
Serve with 1 serving Winning Combo Salad (page 261)

Vegan Burger with Quinoa and Spinach: 1 vegan burger (for
example Fry's brand or Beyond Meat Burger), 125g cooked quinoa
Fresh baby spinach leaves, drizzled with balsamic vinegar or
low-sodium soy sauce

1 vegan burger (for example Fry's brand or Beyond Meat Burger)
1 whole-wheat pitta
Lettuce and sliced tomato, mustard and ketchup
Serve with a mixed green salad drizzled with balsamic vinegar

1 vegan burger (for example Fry's brand or Beyond Meat Burger)
Steamed or roasted green beans, broccoli, cauliflower or asparagus
(unlimited), seasoned with garlic powder, herbs, salt and pepper, or
Miraculous Cauliflower Mash (page 251)
125g cooked brown rice or ½ baked sweet potato

1 baked sweet potato (200g)
1 small or ½ large tin baked beans (200g total)
Mixed green salad, plus diced tomato wedges, seasoned with salt
and pepper, and drizzled with balsamic vinegar

1 large bowl of soup (see recipes starting on page 253)
Serve with 1 wholemeal roll or pitta bread and green side salad

1 vegan burger (for example Fry's brand or Beyond Meat Burger)
Fresh spinach/salad leaves, drizzled with balsamic vinegar
1 serving Quinoa Salad with Avocado, Mango and Pomegranate
(page 247)

1 vegan burger (for example Fry's brand or Beyond Meat Burger)
Fresh spinach/salad leaves, drizzled with balsamic vinegar
1 serving Rainbow Brown Rice Salad (page 262)

1 vegan burger (for example Fry's brand or Beyond Meat Burger)
Fresh spinach/salad leaves, drizzled with balsamic vinegar
1 serving Quinoa Tabbouleh Salad (page 264)

AFTER DINNER OR LATE-EVENING SNACKS

Drink herbal tea, and chooser any of the following snack options –
only if hungry!

* 30g dark chocolate (70 per cent cocoa or above) plus fresh fruit
(1 apple, or pear or orange)
Mug of herbal tea

* Fresh fruit (1 apple, or pear or orange), plus 12 almonds or
cashew nuts
Mug of herbal tea

* Baked Apple with Pecan Nuts: 1 baked apple (or fresh if
preferred), sprinkled with stevia or xylitol and cinnamon, plus 2 tbsp
chopped pecan nuts
Mug of herbal tea

* 150g natural soya yoghurt (unsweetened), plus 75g blueberries
mixed with stevia and cinnamon
Mug of herbal tea

* 25g mixed dried fruit and nuts
Mug of herbal tea

* 30g dark chocolate (70 per cent cocoa or above) plus 75g strawberries or mixed berries
Mug of herbal tea

* 2 vegan oatcakes, plus 2 tbsp (30g) reduced-fat hummus or The Food Effect Spinach Hummus (page 252)
Mug of herbal tea

* Pear with Pecan nuts: serve half a baked pear (or fresh if preferred), sprinkled with stevia and cinnamon, and 2 tbsp crushed pecan nuts
Mug of herbal tea

* Strawberries with Pecan Nuts: 75g sliced strawberries, plus 2 tbsp crushed pecan nuts, top with stevia or xylitol
Mug of herbal tea

* 150g natural soya yoghurt (unsweetened) plus 75g strawberries mixed with stevia and cinnamon
Mug of herbal tea

Apple with Almond Butter: slice 1 apple thinly or into wedges and spread the slices with almond butter (1 level tbsp total)

Apple with Peanut Butter: slice 1 apple thinly or into wedges, and spread the slices with peanut butter (1 level tbsp total)

4 tbsp Sweet-and-Spicy Crunchy Chickpeas (page 265)

1–2 Hummus-Stuffed Dates (page 266)

25g Sweet-and-Spicy Nuts (page 267)

1–2 Dairy-Free 'Ferrero Rocher' Balls (page 267)

1 serving Guilt-Free Chocolate Mousse (page 268)

1–2 Chocolate, Date and Tahini Truffles (page 269)

1–2 All-Healthy Raw Chocolate Truffle Balls (page 269)

1–2 Raw Bakewell Tart Balls (page 270)

1 Chocolate Peanut Cluster, plus 1 serving fresh fruit (page 271)

1 No-Bake Fibre-Filled Brownie Bar (page 271)

1–2 Peanut Cookie Energy Balls (page 272)

1–2 Tropical Mango Energy Balls (page 273)

1 slice Vegan Key Lime Pie (page 274)

CHAPTER 13

The Food Effect Diet Vegan Recipes

Simple, healthy, delicious

In this chapter you'll find all of the recipes specified in both the Attack Phase and Lifestyle Phase of The Food Effect Diet Vegan meal plan and the options given in Chapters 11 and 12. All the recipes are super-simple, quick and easy to prepare, demonstrating that preparing healthy vegan food doesn't require you to spend hours cooking in the kitchen.

For practical purposes, most of the recipes serve one or two people – those recipes that make two portions or more are often included in the plans for the next day's lunch or dinner, so that leftovers can be put to good use (many freeze well, too). Recipes can, of course, also be doubled if you're doing the plan along with a friend or partner, or if you are feeding family or friends.

Non-vegans will love all these recipes just as much too.

* indicates an Attack Phase recipe

BREAKFASTS

* Apple Pie Overnight Oats
* Chocolate Chia Seed Pudding

* Egg-Free Coconut French Toast
* Perfect Porridge
* Avocado Toast
* Blueberry Chia Seed Jam
* Dairy-Free Protein Parfait
Blueberry Bliss Protein Shake
Nutty Vanilla Overnight Oats
Healthy Wholesome Energy Bars
Guilt-Free Courgette Muffins
The Food Effect Green Power Shake
The Food Effect Chocolate Peanut Butter Power Shake
The Food Effect Chocolate Green Power Shake
Sweet Potato Pie Smoothie

LUNCHES AND DINNERS

* Quinoa Salad with Roasted Vegetables
* Avocado and Chickpea Salad
* Roasted Vegetable, Chickpea and Sunflower Seed Salad
* Beetroot Burgers
* Cauliflower and Chickpea Burgers
* Spicy Stuffed Sweet Potato
* Tofu, Spinach and Strawberry Salad with Sweet Poppy
Seed Dressing
* Avocado, Spinach and Strawberry Salad with Sweet Poppy
Seed Dressing
* Protein-Packed Green Skinny Noodle Bowl
* Vegan Cauliflower Cheese
* Vegan Stuffed Pepper
* Teriyaki Tofu
* Vegan Chinese 'Chicken' Stir-Fry
* Chinese-Style Tofu and Kale
* Avocado and Almond Salad
* Slow-Cooker Sweet Potato Vegan Chilli
* Green Bean and Butternut Casserole with Crunchy Peanut Butter Sauce

Pulled Barbecue Jackfruit served with Red Cabbage Slaw
Barbecue Jackfruit Burgers
World Famous Vegetable Tagine
Super-Simple Spaghetti Dish
Quinoa, Wild Rice and Sweet Potato Salad
The New Green Toast
Cauliflower Burger Pitta
Easiest Ever One-Pot Hummus Pasta
Curried Root Vegetable and Lentil Casserole
Quinoa Salad with Avocado, Mango and Pomegranate
Healthy Hearty Minestrone
Protein-Packed Pasta Dish
Vegetable Bolognaise

SOUPS AND SIDE DISHES

* Miraculous Cauliflower Mash
* Miraculous Butternut Squash Mash
* The Food Effect Spinach Hummus
* Dairy-Free Creamy Cauliflower Soup
* Gorgeously Green Soup
Best-Ever Healthy Homemade Hummus
Minted Mushy Peas
Butternut Squash and Apple Soup with Spiced Pumpkin Seeds
The Food Effect World Cup Pea Soup
Easiest-Ever Red Lentil Soup
Carrot, Ginger and Sweet Potato Soup
Fresh Tomato Soup with Mixed Green Pesto
Healthy Hearty Minestrone (see 'Lunches and dinners' for recipe)
Quinoa, Wild Rice and Sweet Potato Salad (see 'Lunches and dinners' for recipe)
Winning Combo Salad
Red Cabbage Slaw
Quinoa Salad with Avocado, Mango and Pomegranate (see 'Lunches and dinners' for recipe)

Rainbow Brown Rice Salad
Quinoa Tabbouleh Salad

SNACKS AND SWEET TREATS

* The Food Effect Spinach Hummus (see 'Side dishes' for recipe)
* Chocolate Chia Seed Pudding (see 'Breakfasts' for recipe)
* Blueberry Chia Seed Jam (see 'Breakfasts' for recipe)
Best-Ever Healthy Homemade Hummus (see 'Side dishes' for recipe)
Healthy Homemade Peanut Butter
Sweet-and-Spicy Crunchy Chickpeas
Hummus-Stuffed Dates
Sweet-and-Spicy Nuts
Dairy-Free 'Ferrero Rocher' Balls
Guilt-Free Chocolate Mousse
Chocolate, Date and Tahini Truffles
Guilt-Free Courgette Muffins (see 'Breakfasts' for recipe)
All-Healthy Raw Chocolate Truffle Balls
Raw Bakewell Tart Balls
Chocolate Peanut Clusters
No-Bake Fibre-Filled Brownie Bars
Raw Peanut Cookie Energy Balls
Tropical Mango Energy Balls
Vegan Key Lime Pie

Note: During the 28-day Attack Phase, follow the specific serving/topping suggestions in the plan in Chapter 11. Once you reach your goal weight (during the Lifestyle Phase), you can be more flexible and creative.

The recipes

Use the recipes in conjunction with the meal plans for the Attack Phase.

Unless otherwise stated in the recipes:

- Vegetables and fruits are medium in size.
- All nuts are shelled and unsalted.
- Herbs are fresh.

BREAKFASTS

Apple Pie Overnight Oats

This tastes just like eating a bowl of apple pie for breakfast, although these oats are totally healthy and waistline-friendly.

Serves 1

40g rolled oats
240ml unsweetened almond milk, plus extra if needed
½ apple, chopped
1 tsp stevia or xylitol
½ tsp ground cinnamon
a pinch of salt
chopped walnuts, mixed seeds or raisins, to serve (optional)

Put all the ingredients in an airtight container or jar. Stir well and leave in the fridge overnight. When ready to eat, remove from the fridge, stir and enjoy. Add a dash more milk if you prefer a thinner consistency. Serve with your choice of chopped walnuts, mixed seeds or raisins, if you like.

Chocolate Chia Seed Pudding

Enjoy this delicious breakfast or healthy sweet treat that can be prepared the night before, ready to grab the next day. Chia seeds are rich in protein and omega-3 fatty acids.

Serves 1

180ml unsweetened almond or cashew milk, plus extra if needed
½ tsp vanilla extract
1 tbsp unsweetened cocoa powder
1 tbsp agave or maple syrup
½ tsp ground cinnamon
3 tbsp chia seeds
blueberries or strawberries, to serve

Put all the ingredients, except the chia seeds, in a bowl or jar. Stir well until the cocoa powder is dissolved. Add the chia seeds and mix well. Leave overnight in the fridge. When ready to eat, stir well before serving. The consistency can be adjusted by adding more milk if you like. Top with blueberries or strawberries and serve.

Egg-Free Coconut French Toast

A 'healthified' vegan version of the classic French toast.

Serves 1

4 tbsp unsweetened almond or coconut milk
½ tbsp wholemeal flour
½ tbsp nutritional yeast flakes
½ tsp granulated stevia/xylitol (or sweetener of your choice), plus extra for sprinkling
a pinch of salt

1 slice of wholemeal bread (or any bread of your choice, such as sourdough, spelt or gluten-free)
unsweetened desiccated coconut, for sprinkling
coconut oil or cooking spray oil, for greasing
ground cinnamon, for sprinkling
mixed berries or strawberries, to serve
agave or maple syrup, to drizzle (optional)

Mix the almond milk, flour, nutritional yeast, sweetener and salt together in a shallow bowl. Dip the bread into the mixture to cover fully. Sprinkle the coconut generously over both sides to coat well.
Grease a non-stick frying pan lightly and heat over a medium heat. Cook the bread on both sides until golden. Transfer to a plate.
Sprinkle generously with stevia and ground cinnamon, then serve with mixed berries and a drizzle of agave syrup, if you like.

Perfect Porridge

This porridge is delicious topped with 1 tbsp of the following: sunflower seeds or pumpkin seeds, flaked almonds, peanut butter or almond butter, plus fresh blueberries, strawberries or mixed berries.

Serves 1

40g porridge oats
180ml unsweetened almond or cashew milk
2 tsp stevia or xylitol
a pinch of salt
ground cinnamon, to taste

Put the oats and milk in a small saucepan over a medium heat. Cook, uncovered, for 5 minutes, stirring as the oats thicken and reach the consistency you like (add a little water if necessary).

Once the oats are cooked and creamy, add the stevia, salt and cinnamon. Stir and remove from the heat. Spoon the porridge into a bowl. Leave to stand for a few minutes before eating – it swells and gets much better. Top with desired toppings as suggested.

Avocado Toast

A classic favourite.

Serves 1

1 small or ½ large ripe avocado
juice of ½ lemon
1 tomato, finely chopped
paprika, to taste
1 slice of wholemeal, rye or sourdough bread
chilli powder or chilli flakes, optional
salt and ground black pepper

Slice the avocado in half and remove the stone. Scoop the flesh into a bowl and mash roughly with a fork, then add the lemon juice. Add the tomato to the bowl. Season generously with salt, pepper and paprika and mix together well.
Toast the bread, then top the toast with the avocado mixture. Sprinkle with chilli powder, if you like, and serve.

Blueberry Chia Seed Jam

This is not your typical jam. Thanks to the chia seeds, it's packed with protein, fibre and healthy omega-3 fatty acids. It makes the perfect topping on toast, or with dairy-free yoghurt, porridge and so much more.

Makes 1 large jar

180g frozen blueberries
2 tbsp agave syrup
¼ cup chia seeds

Put the blueberries into a small saucepan over a medium heat with 2 tsp water and the agave syrup. Simmer for 5 minutes until soft and cooked through.

Mash with a fork or potato masher until well mashed. Stir in the chia seeds, then transfer to a large bowl. Leave to cool fully and leave in the fridge overnight.

Transfer the jam to an airtight jar the next day. Store in the fridge until ready to use, and use within 10 days. Serve as you like (see the plan and meal options for suggestions).

Dairy-Free Protein Parfait

Serves 1

170g dairy-free Greek-style yoghurt
30g porridge oats
75g mixed berries (strawberries, blueberries or blackberries)
½ tsp ground cinnamon
a drizzle of agave syrup (1–2 tsp)

Layer the yoghurt, oats and berries in a large glass or a bowl. Sprinkle with the cinnamon and drizzle with agave syrup. Serve.

Blueberry Bliss Protein Shake

With over 20g of protein, this decadent-tasting smoothie makes a perfect light yet filling breakfast or post-workout snack. With blueberries being the main ingredient, this shake is packed with health benefits: when researchers at Tufts University analysed 60 fruits and vegetables for their antioxidant capability, blueberries rated the highest. They are also a good source of vitamin C, fibre, manganese, vitamin E and riboflavin.

Serves 1

1 scoop (25g) vanilla (or any flavour) vegan protein powder
180ml unsweetened almond milk
130g frozen blueberries
1 handful of ice cubes
generous sprinkle of ground cinnamon
extra stevia or xylitol, to taste (optional)

Put the ingredients into a blender or food processor and whizz until completely smooth. Pour into a large glass and serve.

Nutty Vanilla Overnight Oats

Serves 2

100g porridge oats
240ml unsweetened almond or cashew milk, plus extra to serve, if needed
¼ tsp ground cinnamon
1 tsp stevia or xylitol
½ tsp vanilla extract
a pinch of salt
2 tbsp chopped walnuts, or other nuts of your choice
berries (such as blueberries) and a drizzle of agave syrup, to serve

Put the oats in a bowl and add the milk, cinnamon, stevia, vanilla extract and salt. Stir together well, then cover and leave in the fridge overnight.

In the morning, stir well. Add a splash of extra milk if you prefer a thinner consistency. Top with the walnuts and berries, and a drizzle of agave syrup, and serve.

Healthy Wholesome Energy Bars

These bars are chewy, filling and delicious. They're rich in protein, fibre and heart-healthy monounsaturated fats – a perfect homemade vegan energy bar.

Makes 8 bars

coconut oil or cooking spray oil, for greasing
125g porridge oats (you can use gluten-free oats, if required)
140g almonds
16 pitted Medjool dates (soaked in hot water for 10 minutes, if not soft)
20g unsweetened desiccated coconut
3 tbsp agave syrup or maple syrup
½ tsp almond essence or vanilla extract
a pinch of salt

Preheat the oven to 180°C/Gas 4, and grease a 20cm square baking tin and line it with baking paper. Put the oats and almonds in a food processor and whizz until finely ground. Add the dates, coconut, agave syrup, almond essence and salt, then process again. Slowly add 120ml water while you continue to process the ingredients until a thick, sticky, cohesive batter forms.
Spread the batter evenly in the prepared baking tin and press down well with a spatula so that it is firmly packed. Bake for 20 minutes, then leave to cool. Transfer the baking paper with its contents to a flat surface, then cut into 8 bars.

Guilt-Free Courgette Muffins

These incredibly delicious muffins are full of natural fibre and whole-grain goodness. Courgettes are an excellent weight-friendly food, as they are extremely low in calories, with only 14 calories per 100g. These muffins have a low GI, keeping you fuller for longer and preventing those slumps that you get after eating sugary, high-GI white muffins and baked goods.

Makes 8 muffins

cooking spray oil, for greasing (optional)
210g wholemeal (or spelt) flour
½ tsp bicarbonate of soda
¾ tsp salt
1 tsp ground cinnamon
125g coconut sugar
60ml sunflower oil
115g apple sauce (no added sugar)
60ml unsweetened almond or soya milk
1 tsp apple cider or white vinegar
1 courgette, grated
45g dark chocolate chips
40g raisins

Preheat the oven to 180°C/Gas 4. Grease a non-stick muffin tray with cooking spray, or line with 8 paper or silicone muffin liners. Add the flour, bicarbonate of soda, salt and cinnamon to a bowl and stir in the coconut sugar. Set aside.
In another bowl combine the sunflower oil, apple sauce, milk, vinegar and courgette. Stir the wet ingredients into the dry ingredients. Add the chocolate chips and raisins, then mix until just combined.
Divide the mixture among the muffin cups and bake for 20 minutes. Remove from the oven and leave to cool before removing the muffins from the tin.

The muffins can be stored in an airtight container or plastic ziplock bag for several days at room temperature, or they can be frozen for up to 6 months.

The Food Effect Green Power Shake

A great protein-packed breakfast or post-workout snack.

Serves 1

70g frozen chopped spinach
3 handfuls of small ice cubes
1–2 scoops (30g) vegan protein powder (vanilla or any flavour of choice)
1 tbsp nut butter, such as peanut or almond butter*
1 tbsp granulated sweetener (such as stevia)
1 tsp ground cinnamon
¼ tsp ground ginger (optional)
a few drops of almond essence (optional, but recommended)
120ml unsweetened almond milk

*You can substitute this with ½ an avocado for a nut-free version, if you like.

Put the spinach and ice in a blender or food processor. Whizz until the ice is fully crushed Add the remaining ingredients and whizz for several minutes on the highest speed until smooth. Pour into a large glass and serve.

The Food Effect Chocolate Peanut Butter Power Shake

This shake tastes like a Reese's chocolate in a cup ... except, of course, it's totally vegan.

Serves 1

70g frozen chopped spinach
2 handfuls of small ice cubes
1–2 scoops (30g) vegan protein powder (vanilla or any flavour
of choice)
1 tbsp peanut butter
1 tbsp unsweetened cocoa powder
1–2 tbsp granulated sweetener (such as stevia or xylitol)
1 tsp ground cinnamon
a pinch of salt
120ml unsweetened almond milk

Put the spinach and ice in a blender or food processor. Whizz until
the ice is fully crushed. Add the remaining ingredients, and whizz for
several minutes on the highest speed until smooth. Pour into a large
glass and serve.

The Food Effect Chocolate Green Power Shake

This is so chocolaty and decadent-tasting that you'll have a hard time
believing it's full of so much green goodness.

Serves 1

70g frozen chopped spinach
2 handfuls of small ice cubes
½ avocado
1–2 scoops (30g) vegan protein powder
1 tbsp unsweetened cocoa powder
1–2 tbsp granulated sweetener (such as stevia), to taste
1 tsp ground cinnamon
120ml unsweetened almond milk

Put the spinach and ice in a blender or food processor. Whizz until the ice is fully crushed. Add the flesh of the avocado and the remaining ingredients, and whizz for several minutes on the highest speed until smooth. Pour into a large glass and serve.

Variation: add some peppermint essence and you'll have the most delicious chocolate mint shake.

Sweet Potato Pie Smoothie

I love shakes and also love sweet potatoes, so I've combined the two and come up with this super-simple, sweet and delicious smoothie recipe that's healthy and indulgent, and tastes just like sweet potato pie in a glass.

Serves 1

1 sweet potato, peeled
2 handfuls of ice cubes
120ml coconut water
60ml unsweetened almond or coconut milk
1 heaped tbsp peanut or almond butter
1–2 tbsp agave syrup, to taste
½ tsp vanilla extract
½ tsp ground cinnamon, plus extra for serving
a pinch of salt

Prick the sweet potato with a fork and cook in the microwave for 8–10 minutes, or until completely soft. Leave the sweet potato until cold.
Put the ice in a blender or food processor and whizz until completely crushed. Add the sweet potato and the remaining ingredients, and whizz on high speed until smooth. Pour into a tall glass and dust with extra cinnamon. Serve.

LUNCHES AND DINNERS

Quinoa Salad with Roasted Vegetables

Serves 2

2 small courgettes, peeled and chopped
1 carrot, chopped
1 small red onion, peeled and chopped
380g frozen broccoli or cauliflower
olive oil or cooking spray oil, for roasting
paprika, to taste
130g quinoa, rinsed
juice of 1 lemon, to serve
salt and ground black pepper

Preheat the oven to 180°C/Gas 4. Put the vegetables in a roasting tin and lightly coat with the olive oil. Season well with salt, pepper and paprika, and mix to coat. Roast for 20 minutes or until tender.
Meanwhile, put the quinoa in a saucepan and add 360ml water and a generous pinch of salt. Bring to the boil, then reduce the heat to a simmer, cover and cook for 15–20 minutes or until the water is absorbed and the quinoa is fluffy. Put the quinoa in a large serving dish and add the vegetables, then toss together. Serve warm or at room temperature with lemon juice and salt and pepper to taste.

Avocado and Chickpea Salad

Serves 1

a large serving of mixed salad leaves
½ × 400g tin chickpeas, rinsed and drained

2 spring onions, chopped
½ avocado
paprika, to taste
a pinch of chilli powder or cayenne pepper (optional)
juice of ½ lime or lemon
salt and ground black pepper

Put the salad leaves on a plate. Scatter over the chickpeas and spring onions.

Cut the avocado flesh into thin slices or cubes, and scatter over the salad.

Sprinkle the paprika over the salad, plus a pinch of chilli, if using. To serve, dress with lime juice, and season with salt and pepper.

Roasted Vegetable, Chickpea and Sunflower Seed Salad

Chickpeas are an amazing source of plant-based protein and fibre. Sunflower seeds are rich in vitamin E, an essential fat-soluble vitamin, and are perfect to aid absorption of all the nutrients from these colourful antioxidant-rich vegetables.

Serves 1

2 large handfuls of assorted vegetables cut into chunks (red onions, courgette, red or yellow pepper, mushrooms, aubergine)
1 tsp dried mixed herbs
olive oil or cooking spray oil, for roasting
a large portion of mixed salad leaves or spinach
½ × 400g tin chickpeas, rinsed and drained
1 tbsp sunflower seeds
balsamic vinegar, to drizzle
chopped fresh mixed herbs, such as parsley and coriander
salt and ground black pepper

Preheat the oven to 180°C/Gas 4. Put the vegetables in a roasting tin, sprinkle with the dried mixed herbs and lightly coat with the olive oil. Season well with salt and pepper, and mix to coat.

Roast for 20–30 minutes or until tender and slightly browned. Leave to cool to room temperature or chill in the fridge to use later.

When ready to eat, put the salad leaves on a plate. Add the roasted vegetables. Top with the chickpeas and sunflower seeds. Drizzle with balsamic vinegar, and season with fresh herbs, salt and pepper. Serve and enjoy.

Beetroot Burgers

These veggie burgers are full of protein, fibre and a wealth of vitamins, minerals and antioxidants. Meat eaters will love them just as much, too.

Makes 8 burgers (allow 2 per person)

100g quinoa, rinsed
400g tin red kidney beans, rinsed and drained
3 ready-cooked vacuum-packed whole beetroot, grated
4 tbsp chopped fresh coriander
4 tbsp chopped fresh mint
1 tsp ground cumin
½ tsp chilli powder (optional)
½ tsp paprika
½ tsp sea salt
2 tbsp lemon juice
25g oat flour (see tip), plus extra if needed
olive oil, for brushing
wholemeal pitta, or brown rice or whole-wheat couscous and a green salad, to serve

Put the quinoa in a saucepan and add 300ml water. Bring to the boil then reduce the heat, cover and simmer for 15–20 minutes or until tender and fluffy.

Put the kidney beans in a large bowl and mash well using a fork. Add the beetroot to the bowl along with the cooked quinoa, herbs, spices and salt. Mash well until everything is combined. Stir in the lemon juice and oat flour until combined. The mixture should stick together well. Add more flour if you need a thicker consistency. Chill the mixture in the fridge for 30 minutes or until ready to cook.

Preheat the oven to 190°C/Gas 5. Line a baking tray with baking paper. Form the mixture into eight burgers. Arrange the burgers on the baking tray and brush the tops lightly with oil. Bake for 30–40 minutes, gently turning them over halfway through. Serve in pitta bread with salad (see the plan and meal options for more specific serving suggestions).

Tip: you can make the oat flour by grinding 25g oats in a food processor.

Cauliflower and Chickpea Burgers

Serve these burgers with Red Cabbage Slaw (see page 262) or a fresh green salad, and some brown rice, couscous or quinoa. See also the variation below for an easy, healthy and delicious way to utilise a left-over burger.

Makes 8 burgers (allow 2 per person)

1kg bag frozen cauliflower, defrosted
½ × 400g tin chickpeas, rinsed and drained
2 tbsp Dijon mustard
2 tbsp wholemeal flour or oat flour (see tip)
2 tbsp lemon juice
¼ tsp chilli flakes
a small handful of parsley leaves

2 tbsp capers, drained
120g dried breadcrumbs
olive oil, for greasing
salt and ground black pepper

Preheat the oven to 180°C/Gas 4. Drain the cauliflower completely. Put all but 3 large cauliflower florets in a food processor together with the chickpeas, mustard, flour, lemon juice, chilli flakes and ½ tsp salt. Whizz until smooth, and then transfer to a large mixing bowl.

Put the parsley and capers into the same processor bowl and chop semi-finely. Add the remaining 3 cauliflower florets, but don't process until totally smooth – you want some texture in the cauliflower to remain. Combine this mixture with the chickpea mixture and 40g of the bread-crumbs. Season with salt and pepper.

Line a large baking sheet with baking paper and coat lightly with olive oil. Combine the remaining breadcrumbs with ½ tsp salt and spread out onto a large dinner plate.

Divide the mixture into eight burgers and then coat them in the bread-crumbs and put them on to the prepared baking sheet.

Bake for 15 minutes, then turn them over carefully and bake for another 15 minutes until lightly browned. Remove from the oven and serve warm or at room temperature.

Tip: you can make oat flour by grinding whole oats in a food processor.

Spicy Stuffed Sweet Potato

This dish is perfect served with a mixed green salad.

Serves 1

1 sweet potato (around 250g)
1 tsp olive oil or cooking spray oil

½ red onion, diced
½ × 400g tin kidney beans, rinsed and drained
200g tin chopped tomatoes
1 tbsp tomato purée
½ fresh chilli, deseeded and sliced, or pinch of cayenne pepper or
dried chilli flakes
½ tsp paprika
salt and ground black pepper

Preheat the oven to 190°C/Gas 5 and bake the sweet potato for 1
hour or until soft. (Alternatively, cook in a microwave on Full Power for
8 minutes.)
Heat the oil in a non-stick frying pan over a medium heat and cook the
onion for 5 minutes or until softened. Add the kidney beans, chopped
tomatoes, tomato purée, chilli, paprika, and salt and pepper to taste.
Heat through. Serve piled on the baked sweet potato.

Tofu, Spinach and Strawberry Salad with Sweet Poppy Seed Dressing

A protein-packed sweet and refreshing salad.

Serves 1

150g firm tofu
olive oil or cooking spray oil, for greasing
½ tsp dried mixed herbs
55g baby spinach leaves
75g strawberries, sliced into halves
1 tbsp toasted flaked almonds

Dressing:
1 tbsp lemon juice

1 tbsp white wine vinegar
½ tsp low-sodium soy sauce
½ tsp olive oil
1 tsp stevia or xylitol
½ tsp poppy seeds

Cut the tofu into thick slices. Brush the tofu slices with oil on both sides (or spray with spray oil) and then season them with the herbs, salt and pepper. Cook in a pan on medium-high heat until browned on both sides. Set aside.

Put the dressing ingredients in a small bowl and mix well. Put the spinach leaves and strawberries in a bowl and toss them with the dressing. Add the tofu. Top with the toasted flaked almonds and serve.

Avocado, Spinach and Strawberry Salad with Sweet Poppy Seed Dressing

This recipe is a variation on the one above. The tofu is replaced with avocado, but if you're looking for something a bit more substantial, you can add chickpeas or kidney beans to this recipe, too, once you are in the Lifestyle Phase.

Serves 1

55g baby spinach leaves
75g strawberries, cut in half
1 small or ½ large avocado, flesh sliced or diced
1 tbsp toasted flaked almonds

Dressing:
1 tbsp lemon juice
1 tbsp white wine vinegar
½ tsp low-sodium soy sauce
½ tsp olive oil

1 tsp stevia or xylitol
½ tsp poppy seeds

Put the dressing ingredients in a small bowl and mix well. Put the spinach leaves and strawberries into a bowl and toss them with the dressing. Gently add the avocado. To serve, arrange the mixture on a plate and top with the almonds.

Variation: add 60g tinned chickpeas, rinsed and drained, to the salad, if you like.

Protein-Packed Green Skinny Noodle Bowl

Tasty and waistline-friendly, this Asian-inspired dish is fresh and deliciously satisfying.

Serves 2

100g rice noodles
2 handfuls baby spinach or salad leaves
1 tbsp low-sodium soy sauce, plus extra to serve
1 tsp sesame oil
90g shelled cooked edamame beans
1 small avocado, flesh diced
2 spring onions, sliced
black and white sesame seeds, to sprinkle

Cook the rice noodles according to package instructions. Drain in a colander and leave to cool.
Put the spinach leaves into two bowls. Stir the soy sauce and sesame oil into the noodles, then divide them between the bowls.
Add the edamame beans, avocado and spring onion on top of each bowl. Garnish with a sprinkle of black and white sesame seeds, drizzle with extra soy sauce and serve.

Vegan Cauliflower Cheese

Even my meat-eating hubby adores this supper.

Serves 3 (as a main course)

900g frozen cauliflower, defrosted
1 tbsp olive oil
½ tsp garlic powder
½ tsp onion powder
½ tsp paprika, plus extra for sprinkling
green salad and brown rice, to serve

Vegan cheese sauce:
3 tbsp tahini
190ml unsweetened almond or cashew milk
20g nutritional yeast
¾ tsp fine sea salt
¼ tsp ground black pepper

Preheat the oven to 180°C/Gas 4. To make the sauce, put the tahini in a small bowl and add 3 tbsp of the almond milk. Stir very vigorously, using a spoon, for 1–2 minutes until a thick, creamy paste is formed. Add the remaining milk, the nutritional yeast, salt and pepper, and stir well to combine. Set aside.

Put the cauliflower in a large bowl. Drizzle with the olive oil and add the flavourings. Toss together to coat well. Tip the cauliflower mixture into a baking dish, then cook in the oven for 30 minutes. Remove from the oven and pour over the sauce. Sprinkle liberally with extra paprika. Return to the oven and bake for a further 5–10 minutes until cooked and golden. Serve with a green salad and brown rice.

Vegan Stuffed Pepper

This recipe can easily be doubled to make two portions.

Serves 1

olive oil or cooking spray oil, for greasing
1 onion, chopped
1 garlic clove, crushed
100g vegan soya mince (for example Fry's brand)
200g tin chopped tomatoes
a handful of spinach leaves
½ tsp salt
¼ tsp ground turmeric
1 red pepper, top removed, cored and deseeded
ground black pepper
brown rice and a green salad, to serve

Preheat the oven to 180°C/Gas 4. Lightly oil a saucepan, then add
the onion and garlic and cook for 5 minutes or until the onion is softened. Add the mince and cook for 4 minutes or until cooked through
and broken apart to create a smooth mince mixture.
Add the chopped tomatoes and spinach, stir well and cook for 3
minutes or until the spinach leaves wilt. Season with the salt, turmeric
and black pepper to taste.
Using a small spoon, fill the pepper with the mince mixture. Put the
pepper upright in a small baking dish. Bake for 30 minutes until the
pepper has softened. Serve with brown rice and a fresh green salad.

Teriyaki Tofu

Tofu takes on the flavour of other ingredients and can be quickly trans-
formed into a tasty source of protein to accompany a stir-fry.

Serves 1

180g firm tofu, cut into slices
3 tbsp low-sodium soy sauce
1 tsp olive oil
1 tsp grated fresh ginger
1 tsp agave syrup
stir-fried or roasted vegetables (in minimal oil/spray oil), to serve

Put the tofu in a bowl and add the soy sauce, olive oil, ginger and agave syrup.

Heat a frying pan over a medium-high heat and cook the tofu on both sides for 5 minutes or until golden. Serve with stir-fried or roasted vegetables.

Vegan Chinese 'Chicken' Stir-Fry

Don't feel you need to serve hot vegetables with this dish – a fresh green salad complements it perfectly.

Serves 1

spray cooking oil
100g firm tofu, cut into strips
1 tbsp low-sodium soy sauce
½ fresh chilli, deseeded and finely sliced, or ¼ tsp chilli powder
¼ tsp fresh ginger, grated, or a pinch of ground ginger
100g sugar snap peas, cut in half crossways
brown rice and a green salad, to serve (see the plan/meal options for portion sizes)

Spray a frying pan with spray cooking oil and heat over a medium-high heat. Add the tofu and stir-fry for 2–3 minutes until cooked and golden. Add the soy sauce, chilli, ginger and sugar snap peas. Cook for a further 2 minutes. Serve immediately with the brown rice and a fresh green salad.

Chinese-Style Tofu and Kale

This is so much more delicious and healthier than any Chinese takeout.

Serves 2

1 tbsp smooth peanut butter
4 tbsp low-sodium soy sauce
250g firm tofu, cut into cubes
25g cashew nuts
a little coconut oil or cooking spray oil, for frying
1 tbsp sesame oil
250g kale
1 red chilli, deseeded and thinly sliced
5 tbsp chopped fresh coriander
salt

Mix together the peanut butter with 2 tbsp of the soy sauce until well combined. Put the tofu in a shallow dish and add the peanut butter mixture and stir to coat. Leave to marinate for 1 hour.

Meanwhile, put the cashew nuts in a dry saucepan and toast over a medium-high heat, tossing regularly, for 2–3 minutes or until golden brown. Set aside.

Heat the oil for frying in a frying pan over a medium-high heat and pan-fry the tofu until cooked and golden on both sides.

Heat the sesame oil in a large saucepan. Add the kale and a pinch of salt, then leave it to wilt slightly.

For the dressing, whisk together the remaining 2 tbsp soy sauce with the chilli. Divide the cooked kale, tofu and dressing between two serving bowls. Top with the toasted cashew nuts and fresh coriander, and serve.

Avocado and Almond Salad

Serves 1

1 tsp Dijon mustard
1 tbsp balsamic vinegar
2 large handfuls of spinach leaves
½ avocado, flesh sliced
2 tbsp flaked almonds (toasted, if you like)
1 tbsp dried cranberries
salt and ground black pepper

Put the mustard and balsamic vinegar in a small bowl and mix together, then add salt and pepper to taste, and combine well.
Fill a plate or bowl with the spinach leaves, add the sliced avocado, and top with the almonds and dried cranberries. Drizzle with the dressing and serve.

Slow-Cooker Sweet Potato Vegan Chilli

This delicious vegan chilli is packed with protein, fibre and a wealth of antioxidants from the sweet potato and tomatoes. Even meat eaters will go crazy for this one. You can also cook this in a saucepan if you don't have a slow cooker.

Serves 4

1 red onion, chopped
1 red pepper, deseeded and chopped
4 garlic cloves, crushed
1 tbsp mild chilli powder
1 tbsp ground cumin
¼ tsp ground cinnamon
1½ tsp salt

¼ tsp ground black pepper
2 × 400g tins chopped tomatoes
250g sweet potato, peeled and cut into cubes
2 × 400g tins red kidney beans, rinsed and drained
guacamole (see tip on page 241), sliced spring onions,
sliced radishes, tortilla chips, to serve (once you are in the
Lifestyle Phase)

In a slow cooker, combine the red onion, red pepper, garlic, chilli powder, cumin, cinnamon, salt and black pepper. Add the tinned chopped tomatoes, the sweet potato, beans and 250ml water.

Cover and cook on Low for 8 hours, or on High for 5 hours, until the sweet potato is tender. (Times may vary according to your cooker, so check the sweet potato is soft and adjust accordingly.) Alternatively, if you don't have a slow cooker, put all the ingredients into a large saucepan. Bring to the boil, then reduce the heat to a low simmer and leave to cook for 30–45 minutes until the sweet potato is tender. Add a little more water if needed.

Serve the chilli topped with guacamole, spring onion, radishes and tortilla chips (once you are in the Lifestyle Phase). Leftovers will keep well in the fridge for up to 3 days, or can be frozen.

Green Bean and Butternut Casserole with Crunchy Peanut Butter Sauce

This dish is one of my personal favourites. I absolutely adore both butternut squash and peanut butter, and the combination is both heavenly and healthy.

Serves 4

2 tsp olive oil
2 garlic cloves, crushed
5cm piece fresh ginger, peeled and finely chopped

600g ready-prepared (peeled and chopped) butternut squash chunks
2 tsp low-sodium soy sauce
2 tsp coconut sugar or soft brown sugar
200ml vegetable stock (made from MSG-free vegan stock powder)
100g frozen green beans
2 tbsp crunchy peanut butter
4 spring onions, sliced
chopped fresh coriander, to garnish
basmati rice, to serve

Heat the olive oil in a large saucepan over a medium heat and cook
the garlic and ginger for 2 minutes. Add the butternut squash, soy
sauce, coconut sugar and stock. Cover and simmer for 10 minutes.
Add the green beans, then cook for 5 minutes more or until the squash
and beans are soft. Turn off the heat. Add the peanut butter and stir
for 30 seconds. Stir in the spring onions. Garnish with fresh coriander
and serve on a bed of basmati rice.

Pulled Barbecue Jackfruit

This jackfruit recipe is the perfect vegan substitute for pulled chicken
or pork. It'll fool any meat lover, too. It's delicious paired with my
Red Cabbage Slaw, guacamole and rice, or as a filling for Barbecue
Jackfruit Burgers (see page 240).

Serves 2

410g can jackfruit in water (*not* in syrup), rinsed and drained
½ tbsp olive oil
½ onion, diced
½ tsp paprika
½ tsp chilli powder
½ tsp garlic powder
¼ tsp salt

¼ tsp ground black pepper
125ml barbecue sauce
Red Cabbage Slaw (page 262), guacamole (see tip opposite) and
brown rice or white basmati rice, to serve

Chop the jackfruit into bite-sized chunks and set aside. Heat the oil
in a large frying pan over a medium heat and cook the onion for 10
minutes or until very soft.

Add the jackfruit and all the spices and seasonings to the pan. Toss
well to combine fully. Reduce the heat and let the jackfruit cook for
3 minutes.

Add the barbecue sauce and 125ml water, and stir everything
together well. Leave to simmer gently, covered, for 20 minutes, stirring
every 10 minutes to break down the jackfruit. Take off the lid and cook
for a further 10 minutes. Add 60ml water and stir well.

Turn off the heat and use two forks to shred the jackfruit well (you can
also use a potato masher to help break it down), making it resemble
pulled chicken or pulled pork. Serve with Red Cabbage Slaw, guacamole and rice.

Barbecue Jackfruit Burgers

Serves 2

2 wholemeal rolls or burger buns
a few lettuce leaves, and cucumber and tomato slices
1 batch pulled barbecue jackfruit (see Pulled Barbecue
Jackfruit overleaf)
1 avocado, flesh sliced or mashed (or made into
guacamole – see tip)
lemon juice, to taste
2 tbsp vegan mayonnaise
mixed green salad, to serve
salt and ground black pepper

Fill each roll with lettuce, sliced cucumber and tomato, then top each with half the cooked barbecue jackfruit.

Add some sliced avocado, plus lemon juice, salt and pepper. Top each with 1 tbsp vegan mayonnaise. Serve with a mixed green salad.

Tip: Guacamole

Mash the flesh of 1 avocado and add 2 tsp lemon juice, to taste, 1 finely chopped tomato, a few drops of Tabasco sauce and a generous seasoning of garlic powder, and salt and pepper (to taste). Mix well and serve immediately or refrigerate, covered, until ready to serve.

World-Famous Vegetable Tagine

I grew up in a household that was anything but vegan. Being South African, my family loved meat and chicken (me, less so). It was a rare occasion to have a vegetarian, let alone a vegan meal, so this speciality dish of Mum's was always my favourite. My meat-loving brother and dad always devoured this one too, and now so does my meat-loving husband, so it's definitely a real winner. My mum still makes this often, and when she does, we all request a batch, too.

Serves 6

2 tbsp olive oil
2 onions, roughly chopped
2 garlic cloves, crushed
2 tsp ground cumin
2 tsp ground coriander
2 carrots, sliced
4 sweet potatoes, peeled and cubed
4 courgettes, cut into cubes
400g tin chickpeas, rinsed and drained
400g tin chopped tomatoes
250ml vegetable stock (made from MSG-free vegan stock powder)

a pinch of chilli flakes, or to taste
200g spinach leaves
salt and ground black pepper
whole-wheat couscous, brown rice or basmati rice, to serve

Heat a large saucepan with 2 tbsp oil over a medium heat and cook the onions and garlic until the onion is softened. Add the cumin and coriander, and fry for another 1 minute, stirring.
Add the carrots, sweet potatoes and courgettes, and cook for another 5 minutes. Add the chickpeas, tomatoes and stock. Bring to the boil, then stir well, reduce the heat and simmer for 30 minutes. Add salt, pepper and chilli flakes to taste. Leave to cook for another 30 minutes or until the vegetables are tender.
Add the spinach leaves 5 minutes before serving. Adjust the seasoning. Serve over whole-wheat couscous, brown rice or basmati rice.

Super-Simple Spaghetti Dish

This Italian-inspired pasta dish is easy to make, super-healthy and tastes totally heavenly. Whether you're having friends over for dinner, cooking for your family, or just looking for something for yourself to enjoy, this pasta dish is perfect for all. As well as being vegan and dairy-free, it can be made gluten-free by using brown rice pasta, so this really can cater for everyone.

Serves 4

2 large courgettes
2 tbsp pine nuts
garlic powder, to taste
2 tbsp olive oil, plus extra for drizzling
300g whole-wheat or brown rice spaghetti
zest and juice of 1 lemon
salt and ground black pepper

Preheat the oven to 190°C/Gas 5. Cut the courgette lengthways into long, thin strips using a vegetable peeler. Toast the pine nuts in a dry saucepan until just starting to brown. Remove and set aside.

Line a large baking tray with foil or baking paper. Lay the slices of courgette in a single layer on the tray. Season well with garlic powder, salt and black pepper, then brush over with 1 tbsp of the olive oil. Cook in the oven for 10 minutes or until starting to turn golden, watching them carefully.

Remove the tray from the oven, turn the strips over, then season them as before and brush the other sides with the remaining 1 tbsp oil. Return to the oven and cook for 10 minutes, watching them carefully, until lightly coloured and golden. Remove from the oven.

Meanwhile, bring a large saucepan of salted water to the boil, add the pasta and cook according to the package instructions. Drain in a colander, then transfer to a large serving bowl.

Add the courgette slices along with all the roasting juices from the tray. Add the lemon zest and juice, the pine nuts and a drizzle of oil. Season well with salt and black pepper, and serve hot.

Quinoa, Wild Rice and Sweet Potato Salad

This colourful, vitamin-fuelled, antioxidant and protein-packed salad is guaranteed to be a big hit on any buffet table. It also makes a perfect light lunch. With its hearty wholesome ingredients, it's also the ideal salad for winter when you might prefer something a little more comforting.

Serves 2 as a main course, 4 as a side dish

1 sweet potato, peeled and cut into 2cm chunks
olive oil, for drizzling
130g quinoa, rinsed
80g wild rice, rinsed
a handful of rocket leaves

90g pomegranate seeds
4 spring onions, chopped
a handful of mint leaves, chopped
pistachio nuts, to garnish (optional)
salt and ground black pepper

Dressing:
60ml olive oil
2 tbsp red wine vinegar
½ tsp salt

Preheat the oven to 200°C/Gas 6. Put the sweet potato in a roasting tin and drizzle over a little olive oil, then add a sprinkling of salt and black pepper. Roast for 30–45 minutes until soft and slightly browned. Leave to cool.

Put the quinoa in a saucepan with 375ml water. Bring to the boil, then reduce the heat, cover and simmer for 15–20 minutes until all liquid has been absorbed and the quinoa is fluffy. Leave to cool.

Put the wild rice in a saucepan and add 250ml boiling water, return to the boil and add salt to taste. Reduce the heat, cover and simmer for 45 minutes or until the grains have popped. Drain and leave to cool.

In a salad bowl, combine the cooled rice, quinoa and sweet potato, then add the other salad ingredients. Put the dressing ingredients in a small bowl, add some black pepper, and whisk together, then pour over the salad. Toss well to coat, then serve.

The New Green Toast

I'll always be a lover and advocate of the classic Avo Toast, but, in this recipe, toast says goodbye to avocado and welcomes peas as its new best friend.

Serves 4

4 slices of wholemeal bread (or 8 small slices of
sourdough bread)
1 batch Minted Mushy Peas (see page 256)
salt and ground black pepper
mixed green salad drizzled with balsamic vinegar, and some
vegetable crudités, to serve

Toast the bread. Top each slice of toast or sourdough bread with
a thick layer of Minted Mushy Pea spread. Sprinkle with salt and
pepper. Serve with a mixed green salad drizzled with balsamic
vinegar, and some vegetable crudités for a delicious healthy
brunch or lunch.

Cauliflower Burger Pitta

This is an easy, healthy and delicious way to utilise leftover
Cauliflower and Chickpea Burgers.

Serves 1

1 cooked Cauliflower and Chickpea Burger (page 228)
1 wholemeal pitta bread
2 tbsp mustard
1 tbsp reduced-sugar ketchup
salad leaves, sliced cucumber, tomatoes and red pepper

Use the Cauliflower and Chickpea Burger warm or cold. Cut the pitta
bread in half. Spread the inside of each half pitta with mustard and
ketchup. Fill with salad leaves, cucumber, tomatoes, red pepper and
the Cauliflower and Chickpea Burger patty.

Easiest Ever One-Pot Hummus Pasta

I make this as a regular weeknight supper – as my husband and I absolutely love it.

Serves 2

720ml vegetable stock (made from MSG-free vegan stock powder)
200g whole-wheat or brown rice penne or fusilli pasta
225g store-bought pasta marinara sauce
125g hummus (store-bought or homemade)
fresh spinach leaves, to serve

Put the stock in a saucepan and bring to the boil. Add the pasta, reduce the heat and simmer for 12 minutes over a low heat until most of the liquid is absorbed. Add the marinara sauce, then cook for 2 minutes, stirring. Add the hummus and stir through well. Serve in a bowl on a bed of fresh spinach leaves.

Curried Root Vegetable and Lentil Casserole

Serves 4

2 tbsp olive oil
2 garlic cloves, crushed
1 onion, chopped
700g sweet potatoes, peeled and cut into chunks
2 parsnips, thickly sliced
2 carrots, thickly sliced
1 tbsp curry powder
1 litre vegetable stock (made from MSG-free vegan stock powder)
150g red lentils
1 small handful of coriander, leaves roughly chopped

salt and ground black pepper
unsweetened soya natural yoghurt and wholemeal pitta, to serve

Heat the olive oil in a large saucepan over a medium heat and cook the garlic and onion for 3–4 minutes until softened. Keep stirring to prevent burning. Add the sweet potatoes, parsnips and carrots. Turn up the heat and cook for 6 minutes, stirring, until the vegetables are golden.

Stir in the curry powder, pour in the stock and bring to the boil. Add the red lentils, return to the boil and then reduce the heat. Cover and simmer for 20 minutes or until the lentils and vegetables are tender and the sauce has thickened.

Stir in half the fresh coriander. Season with salt and pepper to taste. Serve in bowls topped with the remaining fresh coriander, 1–2 tbsp of soya yoghurt, and wholemeal pitta bread.

Quinoa Salad with Avocado, Mango and Pomegranate

An incredibly versatile recipe, this salad can be served alongside grilled tofu or vegetable burgers but it is also substantial enough to make a delicious light lunch or dinner. Quinoa is rich in protein, and, with heart-healthy fibre-filled pistachio nuts, avocado and pomegranate seeds, this salad ticks all the nutrition boxes.

Serves 2 as a main course, 4 as a side dish

170g red quinoa, or regular white quinoa, rinsed
1 ripe avocado, flesh diced
1 small ripe mango, peeled and diced
80g pomegranate seeds
20g pistachio nuts
4 spring onions, thinly sliced
a few handfuls of fresh spinach or salad leaves

Dressing:
1 tbsp olive oil
2 tbsp balsamic vinegar
1 tsp sesame oil
2 tsp low-sodium soy sauce

Put the quinoa in a saucepan and add 500ml water and a generous pinch of salt. Bring to the boil, then reduce the heat to a simmer, cover and cook for 15–20 minutes or until the water is absorbed and the quinoa is fluffy. Leave to cool slightly.
Put all the salad ingredients in a large bowl. Put the dressing ingredients in a small bowl and whisk together. Add to the salad, and toss well to coat. Serve.

Healthy Hearty Minestrone

This soup is low in fat and full of vitamins, minerals and nutrients. The protein-packed beans and barley, and the satiety-promoting fibre, combined with nutrient-rich veggies and tomato broth (high in the super-antioxidant lycopene), means that this soup will fill you up, not out.

Serves 4–6

2 tbsp olive oil
1 small onion, chopped
2 garlic cloves, crushed
2 celery sticks, diced
1.9 litres vegetable stock (made from MSG-free vegan stock powder)
400g tin cannellini beans, rinsed and drained
100g barley
4 carrots, diced
2 courgettes, diced
1 tsp dried basil
1 tsp dried oregano

1 tsp salt
¼ tsp ground black pepper
450g tinned chopped tomatoes
crusty bread and vegan Parmesan cheese or nutritional yeast, to
serve (optional)

Heat the oil in a large saucepan over a medium heat and cook the
onion, garlic and celery for 5 minutes or until softened.
Pour in the stock, then add the beans and barley. Bring to the boil,
then reduce the heat and simmer for 1 hour.
Add the carrots, courgettes, herbs, salt and pepper. Simmer, uncovered, for a further 1 hour. Add the tomatoes and simmer for 20
minutes. Serve with crusty bread and a sprinkling of vegan Parmesan
cheese or nutritional yeast, if you like.

Protein-Packed Pasta Dish

Serves 4 as a lunch or light supper

300g whole-wheat fusilli pasta, or brown rice pasta or
chickpea pasta
1 courgette, halved lengthways and thinly sliced
1 red pepper, deseeded and diced
2 large vine tomatoes, cut into chunks
400g tin chickpeas, rinsed and drained
80g pitted black olives, sliced

Dressing:
3 tbsp apple cider vinegar
1 tsp salt
1 tbsp Dijon mustard
3 garlic cloves, crushed
3 tbsp olive oil
a pinch of cayenne pepper (optional but recommended)

Bring a large saucepan of salted water to the boil, add the pasta and cook according to the package instructions. Drain in a colander and set aside.

Put the dressing ingredients in a small bowl and mix well. Put the pasta in a large bowl and add the prepared vegetables, chickpeas and olives.

Toss with the dressing and leave it to stand for about 10 minutes for the flavours to develop before serving. Serve at room temperature, or chill in the fridge and serve cold. Any leftovers make a great lunch the next day.

Vegetable Bolognaise

Here is a healthy, delicious vegan version of the classic favourite.

Serves 4

300g whole-wheat or brown rice spaghetti
1 tbsp olive oil
1 onion, chopped
2 carrots, finely chopped
2 celery sticks, sliced
300g tin cut green beans in water, drained and chopped
400g tin chopped tomatoes
2 tbsp tomato purée
125g mushrooms, chopped
¼–½ tsp cayenne pepper, to taste
salt and ground black pepper
a small handful of parsley, leaves chopped

Bring a large saucepan of salted water to the boil, add the spaghetti and cook according to the package instructions. Drain in a colander. Meanwhile, heat the olive oil in a saucepan over a medium heat and cook the onion for 5 minutes or until softened. Add the carrots, celery and green beans. Stir in the tomatoes, tomato purée, mushrooms and cayenne pepper. Season with salt and pepper to taste.

Bring to the boil, then reduce the heat and simmer for 10 minutes. Stir in the parsley. Serve the Bolognaise on the spaghetti and grind some more black pepper over the top. Serve hot.

SOUPS AND SIDE DISHES

Miraculous Cauliflower Mash

Here is the first of two fantastic low-carb, low-calorie highly nutritious recipes for miraculous mash. As I'm sure you'll know by now, I'm not a fan of cutting out carbs, but these comforting bowls of goodness provide far more goodness and far fewer calories than a big bowl of white potatoes. And, of course, the taste is nothing less than miraculous.

Serves 4

600g frozen cauliflower
2 garlic cloves, sliced
1 tsp salt
1–2 tbsp unsweetened almond or cashew milk, as needed
ground black pepper

Cook the cauliflower and garlic in a large saucepan of boiling water for 20 minutes or until soft. Drain in a colander and tip back into the pan.

Add the salt to the pan and whizz to a purée using a hand-held blender. (Alternatively, use a regular blender or a food processor.) Add the milk as necessary, and whizz again to achieve the consistency of mash that you prefer, but don't allow it to get too thin. Season with black pepper to taste, then serve.

Miraculous Butternut Squash Mash

Here is my second mash recipe, which is a flavoursome, nourishing and brightly coloured staple to accompany so many dishes.

Serves 4

1 large butternut squash, peeled, seeded and cubed
1 tsp salt
½ tsp ground cinnamon, plus extra to serve (optional)
2 tbsp agave or maple syrup, plus extra to serve (optional)
chopped pecan nuts or walnuts, to garnish (optional)

Put the squash in a large saucepan and cover with water. Bring to the boil, then reduce the heat, cover and simmer for 30 minutes or until the squash is completely soft and tender.
Drain in a colander and tip back into the pan. Add the salt, cinnamon and agave syrup to the pan and whizz to a purée using a hand-held blender. (Alternatively, use a regular blender or a food processor.) Serve warmed, garnished with the chopped pecan nuts and extra cinnamon and syrup if you like.

Tip: to peel a butternut squash with ease, place the whole, uncooked squash in a 180°C/Gas 4 oven for 30 minutes. Remove and leave to cool completely, then peel.

The Food Effect Spinach Hummus

Here is a delicious twist on the classic favourite.

Serves 4

100g fresh spinach leaves
400g tin chickpeas, rinsed and drained

2 garlic cloves, peeled and left whole
2 tbsp lemon juice
½ tsp ground cumin
1 tsp salt
¼ tsp ground black pepper
1–2 tbsp olive oil
crackers, crudités or wholemeal pitta bread, to serve

Put all the ingredients, except the oil, into a food processor or blender and add 60ml water. Add 1 tbsp of the oil, then whizz until well combined. Add the remaining oil if the mixture becomes too thick.
Spoon into a dish and chill in the fridge. Serve with crackers, crudités or wholemeal pitta bread. The hummus can be stored in an airtight container in the fridge for up to 5 days.

Dairy-Free Creamy Cauliflower Soup

You'll have a hard time believing this soup is so low in calories and fat, and totally dairy-free.

Serves 8

1 tbsp olive oil
1 large onion, chopped
2 garlic cloves, crushed
900g frozen cauliflower
1½ litres vegetable stock (made from MSG-free vegan stock powder)
1 tsp sea salt
ground black pepper
250ml unsweetened almond or cashew milk
truffle oil, to drizzle
pumpkin seeds or za'atar, to garnish (optional)

Heat the oil in a large saucepan over a medium heat and cook the onion and garlic for 5 minutes or until softened. Add the cauliflower and cook for 5–10 minutes until the cauliflower softens.

Pour over the stock and bring to the boil, then reduce the heat and simmer for about 30 minutes until the cauliflower is soft.

Whizz to a purée using a blender or food processor. Season with the salt and black pepper to taste, and stir in the milk, then reheat until just warm. Ladle into bowls and drizzle with truffle oil. Garnish with pumpkin seeds or za'atar, if you like, and serve.

Variation: stir in 1 tsp ground turmeric and a sprinkling of curry powder when you cook the onions, for a delicious twist on this recipe.

Gorgeously Green Soup

This soup is as gorgeous in taste, texture and appearance as it is good for you.

Serves 2

1 tbsp olive oil
1 small onion, chopped
1 garlic clove, crushed
180g spinach leaves
300g tinned baby carrots, drained
360ml vegetable stock (made from MSG-free vegan stock powder)
½ tsp salt
2 thick brown rice cakes

Heat the oil in a large saucepan over a medium heat and cook the onion and garlic for 5 minutes or until the onion is softened.

Add the spinach, carrots, stock and salt. Bring to the boil, then reduce the heat and simmer for 5 minutes or until the spinach leaves have wilted.

Turn off the heat and add the rice cakes by crumbling them in. Stir well. Leave for 5 minutes to go soggy. Whizz the soup using a hand-held blender or food processor until completely smooth.

Best-Ever Healthy Homemade Hummus

The quantities of ingredients here make quite a small batch, so I always double them if I'm making the hummus for guests (or for the week), and recommend doing so. Leftovers never go to waste in my house.

Serves 4

400g tin chickpeas, rinsed and drained
1 garlic clove
60g tahini
juice of 1 lemon
1 tsp salt
¾ tsp ground cumin
¼ tsp ground black pepper
2 tbsp extra-virgin olive oil
wholemeal pitta, crackers or crudités, to serve (optional)

Put the chickpeas in a blender or food processor and add the garlic, tahini, lemon juice, salt, cumin and pepper. (Alternatively, use a bowl and a hand-held blender.) Whizz for 1 minute or until fully blended. Add the oil and 1 tbsp water, then process again until fully combined and smooth. Add another 1 tbsp water if you prefer a thinner consistency of hummus.

Transfer the hummus to an airtight container and store in the fridge for up to 5 days. Serve with wholemeal pitta, crackers or crudités, or simply eat and enjoy it as is.

Roasted Butternut Squash and Apple Soup with Spiced Pumpkin Seeds

The pumpkin seeds here make a perfect protein-rich snack too.

Serves 8

2 tbsp olive oil
1 large onion, diced
2 green apples, peeled and chopped
½ tsp ground cinnamon
½ tsp ground ginger
¼ tsp chilli powder
1½ tsp salt
2 kg butternut squash, peeled and cut into cubes
2 litres vegetable stock (made from MSG-free vegan stock powder)
salt and ground black pepper

Spiced pumpkin seeds:
1 tbsp extra-virgin olive oil
½ tsp ground cinnamon
½ tsp chilli powder
140g pumpkin seeds

Heat the oil in a large saucepan over a medium heat and add the onion, apples, cinnamon, ginger, chilli powder and salt. Cook, stirring occasionally, for 5 minutes. Add the squash to the saucepan, stir to coat and cook for 5 minutes.

Add the stock and bring to the boil, then reduce the heat and simmer, covered, for 40–50 minutes until the squash is soft. Season with salt and pepper.

Allow the soup to cool a little, then whizz until completely smooth using a hand-held blender. (Alternatively, use a regular blender or a food processor.)

To make the spiced pumpkin seeds, put the oil in a small bowl and add the cinnamon and chilli powder. Season with salt and pepper, and mix well together.

Add the pumpkin seeds and stir to coat. Heat a pan over a medium heat. Add the pumpkin seeds and toast in the pan, stirring regularly, for 3–5 minutes until golden. Remove from the heat and leave to cool. Serve the soup hot, with a generous sprinkling of spiced pumpkin seeds on top.

Minted Mushy Peas

I love this dish for brunch or lunch (perhaps paired with some soup and a wholemeal roll), and if you serve it with some seeded crackers or on mini toasts you've got a quick, easy and impressive vegan appetiser, too.

Serves 4

500g frozen peas
3 tbsp olive oil
6 mint leaves
salt and ground black pepper

Put the frozen peas in a bowl and cover with boiling water, then leave for 5 minutes to defrost. Drain the peas and then run them under cold water to refresh them and keep the colour bright green. Drain in a colander, shaking off as much excess water as possible.

Reserve about 3 tbsp of the peas. Put all the remaining peas into a saucepan, and add the olive oil and 2 tbsp water. Cook over a medium heat until all the water has evaporated and the peas are cooked through.

Allow the peas to cool completely, then put them into a blender or food processor and whizz to a purée. While blending, add the mint leaves, a generous pinch of salt, and black pepper to taste. Stir in the reserved whole peas and serve. Delicious as a side dish, on sourdough bread, or healthy wholegrain toast. See The New Green Toast recipe on page 244.

The Food Effect World Cup Pea Soup

This creamy, yet light and refreshing soup recipe was born out of a dinner party I organised without realising that the timing clashed with a football World Cup final. Thankfully, it was a great success, with guests proclaiming it one of the best soups they'd ever tasted (one football fanatic even said it was worth missing the final for). I serve it with fresh sourdough bread and top it with pumpkin seeds, but you could try some of the other suggestions outlined below, if you like.

Serves 4–6

2 tbsp olive oil
1 large onion, chopped
800ml vegetable stock (made from MSG-free vegan stock powder)
15g fresh mint leaves
800g frozen peas
1 head of romaine or cos lettuce, torn into shreds
2 tsp salt
½ tsp ground black pepper
pumpkin seeds or chopped toasted cashew nuts and chopped chives or mint leaves, to garnish

Heat the oil in a large saucepan over a medium heat and cook the onion for 5 minutes or until softened. Add the stock, mint leaves and peas. Bring to the boil and simmer for 15 minutes.
Add the lettuce, salt and pepper, then simmer for another 10 minutes. Whizz the soup, using a hand-held blender, until smooth and thick. Serve hot, garnished with the seeds, nuts and herbs.

Easiest Ever Red Lentil Soup

Quick, easy, healthy and delicious, this one-pot recipe doesn't even require blending.

Serves 4–6

2 tsp olive oil
1 onion, chopped
2 garlic cloves, crushed
1 tsp ground cumin
300g red lentils, rinsed
1.4 litres vegetable stock (made from MSG-free vegan stock powder)
2 tbsp lemon juice
salt and ground black pepper
chopped fresh coriander, to garnish (optional)

Heat the oil in a saucepan over a medium heat and cook the onion and garlic for 5 minutes or until soft. Add the cumin and cook for 1 minute. Stir in the lentils.
Add the stock and season with salt and pepper. Bring to the boil, then reduce the heat, cover and simmer until the lentils are soft and tender and the soup is beginning to thicken (about 30–40 minutes). Stir in the lemon juice. Adjust the seasoning and serve sprinkled with coriander, if you like.

Carrot, Ginger and Sweet Potato Soup

Serves 4

1 tbsp coconut oil
1 large onion, chopped
2.5cm piece fresh ginger, peeled and chopped
7 carrots, thickly sliced
1 large sweet potato, peeled and cubed
1 litre vegetable stock (made from MSG-free vegan stock powder)
salt and ground black pepper
chopped fresh coriander, chilli flakes, pumpkin seeds or toasted flaked almonds, to garnish (optional)

Heat the oil in a large saucepan over a medium heat and cook the onion and ginger for 5 minutes or until soft. Add the carrots and sweet potato, and cook over a low heat for 15 minutes or until slightly tender. Stir in the stock. Bring to the boil, then reduce the heat, cover and simmer for 30–40 minutes until the sweet potato is soft. Once fully cooked, turn off the heat and whizz the soup using a hand-held blender until completely smooth. Add salt and pepper to taste and serve sprinkled with any of the garnishes listed above, if you like.

Fresh Tomato Soup with Mixed Green Pesto

Low in fat and deliciously satisfying, this soup is full of fibre, vitamins and antioxidants. The addition of spinach and basil pesto gives extra flavour as well as a wealth of nutritional goodness.

Serves 4

1½kg large ripe tomatoes, cut in half horizontally
2 tbsp olive oil, plus extra to drizzle
1 tsp dried oregano
1 onion, chopped
2 garlic cloves, crushed
1 large carrot, chopped
1 celery stick, chopped
480ml vegetable stock (made from MSG-free vegan stock powder)
2 tsp tomato purée
1 tsp stevia or xylitol
salt and ground black pepper

Pesto:
100g baby spinach leaves
100g basil leaves
120g walnuts
2 garlic cloves

½–1 tsp sea salt, to taste
5 tbsp olive oil

Preheat the oven to 200°C/Gas 6 and line a baking tray with baking paper. Put the tomatoes cut-side up on the prepared baking tray. Drizzle with some oil, and sprinkle with the oregano, then season with salt and pepper. Cook in the oven for 45 minutes or until the tomatoes are soft and a bit charred.

Meanwhile, heat the 2 tbsp oil in a large pan over a medium heat and cook the onion, garlic, carrot and celery, stirring frequently, for 6 minutes or until softened.

Add the baked tomatoes and all the juices from the pan to the onion mixture, together with the vegetable stock, tomato purée and xylitol or stevia. Simmer for 30 minutes or until all the vegetables are soft.

While the vegetables are cooking, make the pesto. Whizz the spinach, basil, walnuts, garlic and some salt in a blender or mini food processor to a purée, then slowly add the oil to make a smooth paste. Adjust the seasoning and add a bit of water if the mixture is too thick. Set aside.

Leave the soup to cool a little, then whizz until smooth, using a handheld blender or food processor. Season to taste with salt and pepper. Serve the soup drizzled with the pesto. The pesto can be frozen in ice-cube trays and used when needed, if you like.

Winning Combo Salad

This vibrant, nutritious salad is colourful, eye-catching and delicious.

Serves 4

200g raw beetroot, grated
2 large carrots, grated
340g tin sweetcorn, drained
300g frozen peas, thawed
salt and ground black pepper

Dressing:
2 large ripe tomatoes
2 tbsp agave syrup
4 tbsp extra-virgin olive oil
1 tbsp low-sodium soy sauce

Combine all the salad ingredients in a large bowl.
Whizz the dressing ingredients together using a hand-held blender
or food processor. Pour over the salad and toss through well. Season
with salt and pepper to taste. Cover and chill in the fridge until
ready to serve.

Red Cabbage Slaw

Serves 4

200g red cabbage, core removed
120ml apple cider or malt vinegar
4 tbsp agave syrup
2 tsp salt

Shred the cabbage very finely using a food processor, a mandoline or
a sharp knife. Tip into a large bowl.
In a small bowl, mix the vinegar, agave syrup and salt until well combined. Pour over the cabbage and stir well. Set aside and leave for at
least 1 hour. Stir well before serving.

Rainbow Brown Rice Salad

This colourful substantial salad is guaranteed to go down a treat on
any buffet table. Leftovers also make a great packed lunch, with some
salad leaves added. This dish is low in fat, high in fibre and full of
vitamins, minerals and protein.

Serves 8 as a side dish

50g cashew nuts
6 tbsp mixed seeds (such as sunflower, pumpkin and sesame seeds)
450g brown rice
1 tsp salt
6 spring onions, white parts only, thinly sliced
1 red pepper, deseeded and diced
1 orange pepper, deseeded and diced
60g currants or raisins
3 tbsp fresh chopped parsley
325g tin sweetcorn, drained

Dressing:
2 tbsp olive oil
6 tbsp low-sodium soy sauce
2 tbsp lemon juice
1 large garlic clove, crushed
a generous pinch of sea salt
¼ tsp black pepper
½ tsp dried ginger, or 2.5cm piece fresh ginger, peeled and
finely chopped
½ tsp chilli powder (optional)

Preheat the oven to 180°C/Gas 4. Put all the dressing ingredients in
a small bowl and mix well.
Put the cashew nuts and mixed seeds on a baking tray and toast
in the oven until golden (keep a good eye on them, as they burn
quickly). Remove from the oven and leave to cool. (This step can be
done in advance, and the cashew nuts and seeds can be cooled and
stored in an airtight container or plastic ziplock bag.)
Pour 950ml of boiling water into a saucepan and add the rice
and salt. Bring to the boil, then reduce the heat and simmer for
40 minutes or until the water is fully absorbed and the rice is soft
and cooked.

Drain in a colander, then add the dressing to the rice while it is still warm. Stir to combine, then transfer to a serving bowl and leave to cool completely. Add the remaining ingredients to the rice at least 1 hour before serving. Mix well. Serve either at room temperature, or chilled from the fridge.

Quinoa Tabbouleh Salad

This is delicious as a side dish, or topped with chickpeas, olives and avocado, or pan-fried tofu, for a delicious light lunch or dinner.

Serves 4 as a side dish

170g quinoa, rinsed
½ tsp salt
2 tomatoes, diced
1 small cucumber, diced
½ small red onion, finely chopped
a large handful of flat-leaf parsley, leaves finely chopped
juice of 1 lemon
60ml olive oil
salt and ground black pepper

Put the quinoa in a saucepan and add 480ml water and the salt. Bring to the boil, then reduce the heat to a simmer, cover and cook for 15 minutes or until the water is absorbed and the quinoa is cooked but still a little firm. Remove from the heat and leave to cool.
Add the tomatoes, cucumber, onion and parsley. Dress with the lemon juice and olive oil, and season generously with salt and pepper. Toss together well. Serve at room temperature or chill and serve cold from the fridge.

SNACKS AND SWEET TREATS

Healthy Homemade Peanut Butter

This is an all-natural alternative to store-bought peanut butter.

Makes 1 large jar

450g roasted skinless peanuts
a generous pinch of sea salt (omit if using salted peanuts)
1–2 tbsp agave syrup, to taste

Put the ingredients in the bowl of a high-powered food processor such as a Nutribullet or Vitamix. Whizz until the nuts break down to form a completely smooth, creamy, peanut butter consistency, stopping at intervals to scrape down the sides of the processor. This process does take some time (about 10 minutes, depending on the power of your processor), so do be patient and don't think that it hasn't worked – the nuts go from crushed, to fine crumbs, to a course dough-ball, but then eventually break down to a perfect peanut butter consistency.
Once completely smooth, pour into a sealable jar and store in the fridge for up to 4 weeks – if it hasn't all been eaten by then!

Sweet-and-Spicy Crunchy Chickpeas

A super-delicious fibre-filled protein snack. These chickpeas also make a great topping for hummus, salads or soups.

Makes 4 servings

400g tin chickpeas, drained and rinsed
1 tbsp olive oil

1 tsp paprika
1 tsp chilli powder
½ tsp ground cumin
a pinch of salt
1 tsp agave syrup

Preheat the oven to 180°C/Gas 4 and line a baking tray with baking paper. Put the chickpeas in a bowl lined with kitchen paper, and pat them dry to remove as much of the liquid as possible. Tip the chickpeas into a clean bowl. Add the oil, paprika, chilli powder, cumin and salt, and mix together well to coat.

Spread the chickpeas out on the prepared baking tray and roast for 10 minutes or until just starting to turn golden. Remove from the oven and drizzle with the agave syrup. Return to the oven for a further 5–10 minutes until golden and crisp. Leave to cool completely on the baking tray before transferring to a serving bowl or airtight container. These keep well in an airtight container for up to 1 week.

Hummus-Stuffed Dates

A great snack or post-dinner dessert, these dates will satisfy those sweet cravings healthily, with the added bonus of protein and fibre.

Makes 10 servings

10 large, soft Medjool dates
1 tsp ground cinnamon
250g hummus (shop-bought or homemade)
10 walnut halves

Slice the dates lengthways and remove the stones. Stir the cinnamon into the hummus. Put 2 heaped teaspoons of hummus into each date. Top each with a walnut half. Serve and enjoy.

Sweet-and-Spicy Nuts

Makes 8 servings

¼ tsp cayenne pepper
4 tbsp agave syrup
1 tsp ground cinnamon
¼ tsp ground cumin
1 tsp salt
240g cashew nuts, or almonds or walnuts (or any
combination of these)

Preheat the oven to 180°C/Gas 4 and line a baking tray with baking
paper. Put all the ingredients, except the nuts, into a mixing bowl and
stir together. Add the nuts and stir well to coat evenly.
Spread the nuts in a single layer over the prepared baking tray and
bake for 15 minutes or until browned (making sure they don't burn).
The nuts will be very sticky when they come out of the oven, but they
will crisp up once cooled. Leave to cool completely. Break apart any
clusters. Store in an airtight container in the fridge.

Dairy-Free 'Ferrero Rocher' Balls

These amazing little sweet treats are a healthy vegan version of my
favourite Ferrero Rocher balls. They freeze well and I like to keep a
batch in stock so that healthy snacks are always at hand.

Makes 15–18 balls

200g pitted Medjool dates (soaked in hot water for 10 minutes,
if not soft)
25g unsweetened cocoa powder
130g hazelnuts (you can use roasted)
60g cashew nuts (or an extra 60g hazelnuts)

¼ tsp salt

2 tsp vanilla extract

2 tbsp agave syrup

200g dark chocolate (to coat or drizzle over), broken into pieces, and/
or 130g finely chopped hazelnuts, for rolling and decorating (optional)

Put all the ingredients, except the chocolate and nuts for rolling, into
a food processor and whiz for a few minutes until a thick dough-like
mixture is formed, but there is still some fine texture from the nuts. Keep
scraping down the sides of the processor to incorporate all the dry
ingredients. Transfer the dough mixture to a bowl.

Scoop into 1 heaped tablespoon-sized portions and roll into smooth
balls using your hands.

If coating and decorating the balls, melt the chocolate in a heatproof
bowl over a pan of gently simmering water, making sure the base of
the bowl doesn't touch the water. Put the chopped nuts in a bowl.

Dip each ball into the melted chocolate to coat and then roll it in the
chopped nuts. Put on to a small tray and leave in the fridge to firm for
at least 30 minutes before serving.

Guilt-Free Chocolate Mousse

This tastes exactly like a rich, decadent, unhealthy chocolate mousse,
which is often made with raw eggs. This vegan-friendly version is totally
healthy. The recipe serves four people but can easily be doubled.

Serves 4

2 large very ripe (soft) avocados

25g unsweetened cocoa powder

4 tbsp agave or maple syrup

1 tsp vanilla extract

a pinch of salt

3–4 tbsp unsweetened almond or cashew milk

Scoop out the flesh from the avocados and put it into a blender or food processor. Add the remaining ingredients, except the milk. Add 3 tbsp of the milk and whizz until completely smooth. Add more milk if the mixture is too thick. Spoon into four small ramekins. Chill in the fridge for at least 4 hours, or until ready to serve.

Chocolate, Date and Tahini Truffles

Makes 18–20 balls

270g soft Medjool dates, pitted
40g cashew nuts
95g tahini
1 tbsp unsweetened cocoa powder, plus extra for dusting
¼ tsp salt

Line a plate or small tray with baking paper. Put the dates, cashew nuts, tahini, cocoa powder and salt in a food processor and whizz until finely chopped and well combined. Using slightly damp hands, roll table-spoons of the mixture into balls and dust with the extra cocoa powder. Put on the prepared plate. Leave for 30 minutes in the refrigerator to set. Store in an airtight container in the fridge or freezer until ready to serve.

All-Healthy Raw Chocolate Truffle Balls

These truffle balls freeze well and are one of my all-time favourites.

Makes 15–18 balls

265g pitted Medjool dates (soaked in hot water for 10 minutes, if not soft)
25g unsweetened cocoa powder
70g unsalted almonds or cashew nuts

70g walnuts or peanuts
¼ tsp salt
2 tsp vanilla extract
75g unsweetened desiccated coconut (for rolling) and/or goji berries to decorate (optional)

Put all the ingredients, except the coconut, in a food processor and whizz for a few minutes until a thick dough-like mixture is formed, but there is still some fine texture from the nuts. Keep scraping down the sides of the processor to incorporate all the dry ingredients. Transfer the dough mixture to a bowl.

Scoop into 1 heaped tablespoon-sized portions and roll into smooth balls with your hands. If decorating the balls, put the coconut in a shallow bowl and roll the moist dough balls in it to fully cover them. Put on to a small tray and leave in the fridge for at least 30 minutes before serving.

Raw Bakewell Tart Balls

These balls freeze well and are handy for healthy snacks. They taste so good it's hard to believe that they're all natural and good for you, too.

Makes 15–18 balls

150g cashew nuts
175g pitted Medjool dates (soaked in hot water for 10 minutes, if not soft)
40g raisins
40g dried cranberries
½ tsp vanilla extract
½ tsp almond essence
¼ tsp salt

Put all the ingredients in a food processor and whizz for a few minutes until a thick dough-like mixture is formed, but there is still some fine texture from the nuts. Keep scraping down the sides of the processor to incorporate all the dry ingredients. Transfer the dough mixture to a bowl. Scoop into heaped tablespoon-sized portions, and roll into smooth balls using your hands. Put on to a small tray and leave in the fridge for at least 30 minutes before serving.

Chocolate Peanut Clusters

Quick and easy to make, these no-bake snacks require just a few ingredients. They're tempting and dangerously delicious, but full of goodness – the perfect homemade treats.

Makes a generous batch

325g dark chocolate, broken into pieces, or dark chocolate chips
225g roasted peanuts (you can use salted)
a pinch of salt (if using unsalted peanuts)

Line a large baking tray with baking paper or foil and set aside. Melt the chocolate in a heatproof bowl over a pan of gently simmering water, making sure the base of the bowl doesn't touch the water. Stir and remove from the heat.
Add the peanuts to the chocolate and stir well until they are fully mixed in and coated. Spoon heaped tablespoon-sized portions of the mixture on to the prepared baking tray. Leave to cool, then put in the fridge and leave to set for several hours. The clusters can be stored in an airtight container in the fridge or freezer for several weeks.

No-Bake Fibre-Filled Brownie Bars

Decadent, filling and delicious, these brownie bars are super-healthy, all-natural and perfect when you want something sweet but also want to stick to your healthy-eating habits.

Makes 8 bars

115g almonds, cashew nuts or peanuts (or use a mixture)
20g unsweetened desiccated coconut
175g pitted Medjool dates (soaked in hot water for 10 minutes, if not soft)
65g soft prunes
2 tbsp unsweetened cocoa powder
¼ tsp salt
2–3 tbsp agave syrup

Line a small loaf tin with baking paper. Whizz the nuts in a food processor until finely ground. Add the remaining ingredients to the processor, and whizz for a few minutes until a thick dough-like mixture is formed.

Put the mixture in the prepared tin, and press down firmly. Put it in the fridge for at least 2 hours then remove from the tin and cut into bars or slices. Store in the fridge or freezer (allow time to defrost the bars when you want to eat them).

Peanut Cookie Energy Balls

Looking for the perfect snack to have on hand for those mid-afternoon munchies or late-night sweet cravings? These all-healthy energy balls are just the thing.

Makes 15–18 balls

140g roasted, salted peanuts
265g pitted Medjool dates (soaked in hot water for 10 minutes, if not soft)
50g porridge oats (use gluten-free if required)
1 tsp ground cinnamon
¼ tsp ground ginger (optional)

1 tsp vanilla extract
¼ tsp salt

Put all the ingredients in a food processor and whizz for a few minutes until a thick dough-like mixture is formed. Keep scraping down the sides of the processor to incorporate all the dry ingredients. Transfer the mixture to a bowl.

Scoop into heaped tablespoon-sized portions and roll into smooth balls with your hands. Put on to a small tray and leave in the fridge for at least 30 minutes before serving.

Tropical Mango Energy Balls

These freeze well and make a great tropical-tasting snack.

Makes about 18 balls

125g dried mango
150g cashew nuts
115g pitted Medjool dates (soaked in hot water for 10 minutes, if not soft)
½ tsp vanilla extract
a pinch of ground turmeric
¼ tsp salt
unsweetened desiccated coconut, for rolling (optional, but recommended)

Soak the mango in hot water for 10–15 minutes until soft. Drain in a colander.

Put all the ingredients, except the coconut, in a food processor and whizz for a few minutes until a thick dough-like mixture is formed. Keep scraping down the sides of processor to incorporate all the dry ingredients. Transfer the mixture to a bowl.

Scoop into heaped tablespoon-sized portions and roll into smooth balls using your hands.

If decorating the balls, put the coconut in a shallow bowl and roll the moist balls in it to fully cover them. Put on to a small tray and leave in the fridge for at least 30 minutes before serving.

Vegan Key Lime Pie

A healthy, yet decadent-tasting dessert, this vegan version of a classic will please vegans and non-vegans alike.

Serves 8

For the base:
140g cashew nuts
120g pitted Medjool dates (soaked in hot water for 10 minutes, if not soft)
1 tbsp agave syrup
a pinch of salt

For the filling:
4 large ripe avocados
100g coconut oil
4 tbsp agave syrup
80g coconut sugar (or brown sugar)
juice of 3 limes
a pinch of salt

To decorate:
2 limes, thinly sliced
chopped pistachio nuts
unsweetened desiccated coconut
zest of 1 lime

Line a 20cm cake tin with clingfilm. In a food processor, whizz together the cashew nuts, dates, agave syrup and salt for a few minutes until a thick dough-like mixture is formed but there is still some fine texture from the nuts.

Press the mixture evenly into the base of the prepared cake tin and allow it to come up the sides slightly around the side of the tin. Freeze for 20–30 minutes to set.

To make the filling, put the avocado flesh in a blender or food processor and add the remaining filling ingredients. Whizz, pausing to scrape down the sides as necessary, until you achieve a creamy smooth mixture.

Remove the tin from the freezer and pour the avocado lime mixture on top. Smooth with a spatula and return to the freezer to set for at least 2 hours or overnight.

Decorate with lime slices and pistachio nuts, a sprinkling of coconut and lime zest. Leave to defrost for 30–60 minutes before serving.

CHAPTER 14

Vegan Kitchen Staples and Tips

To ensure your healthy lifestyle changes last

By now you should be familiar with The Food Effect way of eating but, to make it easier, I've compiled a basic list of the main food staples you'll need for the Attack and Lifestyle phases. At the end of the chapter you'll find my tips for making your healthy lifestyle changes last.

Vegan kitchen staples

Keep a selection of the following in your storecupboard, fridge and freezer, to ensure that healthy vegan meals or snacks can always be put together in a matter of minutes. Of course, this is just a guide for you to use and adapt according to your own individual taste, preferences and lifestyle.

Fresh fruit and vegetables

- Apples
- Avocados

- Blueberries
- Carrots, pre-cut carrot sticks or whole carrots
- Cucumber
- Oranges
- Pears
- Spinach, salad leaves
- Sweet potatoes
- Tomatoes, cherry tomatoes

Whole grains and pulses

- Basmati rice
- Brown rice
- Lentils (such as dried red lentils and tinned lentils)
- Oats (porridge oats or rolled oats)
- Quinoa
- Red lentil or chickpea pasta
- Ryvita, brown rice cakes, vegan oat cakes, Corn Thins
- Whole-wheat couscous
- Whole-wheat or brown rice pasta
- Whole-wheat pitta bread
- Wholemeal, rye or sourdough bread

Nuts and seeds

- Almonds, whole and flaked
- Cashew nuts
- Coconut – desiccated coconut (unsweetened)
- Peanut or almond butter (no added sugar)
- Peanuts
- Pistachio nuts
- Pumpkin seeds
- Sesame seeds
- Sunflower seeds
- Walnuts

Dried fruit

- Apricots
- Dates
- Prunes
- Raisins

Tinned foods

- Cannellini beans
- Chickpeas
- Corn
- Jackfruit (in water or brine)
- Lentils
- Peas
- Red kidney beans
- Tomatoes, chopped

Oils, vinegars and condiments

- Apple cider vinegar
- Balsamic vinegar
- Coconut oil
- Extra-virgin olive oil (for drizzling and dressings)
- Ketchup (Heinz: reduced salt and sugar)
- Lemon juice
- Marmite
- Mustard
- Olive oil (for cooking)
- Soy sauce (low-sodium)
- Tahini

Dried herbs and spices etc

- Black pepper
- Cayenne pepper
- Chilli powder
- Cinnamon
- Coriander
- Cumin
- Curry powder
- Dill
- Garlic powder
- Ginger
- Nutritional yeast (with added vitamin B12)
- Paprika
- Salt (fine sea salt)
- Turmeric
- Vegetable stock (MSG-free)

Sweeteners

- Agave syrup
- Cinnamon
- Cocoa powder
- Maple syrup
- Stevia or xylitol (granulated)

Fridge

- Almond, cashew, hemp or oat milk (unsweetened)
- Dairy-free natural yoghurts (for example soya or almond milk yoghurts)
- Hummus (reduced-fat)
- Tofu (firm/extra-firm)
- Vegan falafel balls or burgers, store-bought (for example GOSH Free From brand)

Freezer

- Broccoli
- Cauliflower
- Edamame beans
- Green beans
- Peas
- Sliced bread: wholemeal, rye or sourdough
- Sweetcorn, corn on the cob
- Vegan burgers (for example Fry's brand or Beyond Meat Burger)
- Whole-wheat pitta

Essential extras

- Coffee
- Dark chocolate (70 per cent cocoa or above)
- Herbal teas, green tea

A reminder of The Food Effect basics

You might not immediately remember or follow every single thing that I've recommended throughout this whole book (as the saying goes, 'Rome wasn't built in a day'), but I do strongly advise that you follow, and stick to from the start, my fundamentals for healthy eating and weight loss and The Food Effect Diet Vegan rules. Here they are as a reminder:

The principles in brief

Eat whole, natural foods Avoid packaged, processed foods as much as possible. This means eating whole, natural foods that are close to, if not in, their natural state; for example fresh fruit, vegetables, whole grains, nuts, seeds, beans, chickpeas and lentils. The shorter the list of ingredients on a package of food, the better it is. Nowadays there is an ever-increasing amount of vegan snacks, treats, cheeses and ready meals, with more becoming available. While this is great, they are not always healthy – so check labels and don't be fooled by a label just because it states 'vegan'.

Make sure you never get too hungry Long gaps between meals disrupt your blood-sugar levels, leading to excessive hunger, cravings and, often, stress eating. The outcome is that when you do eventually eat, you're so hungry that it takes a lot more food to feel satisfied, and it's unlikely that you'll binge on celery sticks or apples. Eating small, healthy snacks between meals will help keep your blood sugar stable and your metabolism going strong. The suggested snacks in the meal options will guide you.

Stay well hydrated Often when we think we're hungry we're actually just thirsty. Water aids weight loss by keeping your cells functioning at their fat-burning best, and it also helps your kidneys to flush out excess toxins and chemicals, which may be slowing down your metabolism. Make sure you drink plenty of water throughout the day, as well as one to two glasses before every meal or snack you have.

Slow down your eating and enjoy your food Focus on the food you're eating and don't wolf it down. Avoid eating dinner in front of the TV or lunch in front of your computer. Take time out to enjoy your meal and pay attention to what you're eating. This will ensure that your brain registers when you've eaten enough food, before it's too late.

Eat healthy fats – don't go fat-free This means eating good, healthy unsaturated fats found in nuts, peanut butter, avocados, olive oil and various other healthy oils. Incorporating good fats into your diet will help reduce sugar cravings, increase energy levels and keep you fuller for longer. Whereas too much fat can cause weight gain, too little of the right fats prevents your cells from functioning properly, which affects fat metabolism, hormone balance and energy – all leading to weight gain.

Don't shun carbs Instead, stick to whole-grain, unrefined carbohydrates such as oats, wholemeal or rye bread, brown rice, sweet potatoes and quinoa. Slow-release carbs from whole-grain sources will give you the get-up-and-go you need to stay active and full of energy, while keeping your metabolism going strong all day (and night). They are also great sources of fibre and various other essential nutrients, including the B vitamins niacin, thiamine and folate, and minerals such as zinc, iron, magnesium and manganese.

Know yourself and be realistic Each of us has different needs, goals and preferences, combined with different body types and genetic make-up. You have to recognise your individual needs and be realistic about the changes you can make; for example, if you enjoy having your evening snack late at night, there's no point trying to force yourself to eat it earlier in the day. Evidence has refuted the myth that calories eaten late at night are worse, and has proven that a calorie is a calorie is a calorie. Whether you eat it at 7pm or midnight, there's no difference weight wise; it's your overall daily consumption that counts, which is why you're allowed an evening snack every night.

Eat a rainbow Whether they are fresh, frozen or tinned – try to increase and vary your intake of fruit and vegetables, which, thankfully, being vegan definitely encourages. You'll feel so much better and your body will benefit from all the added vitamins, nutrients, antioxidants and fibre. Diets rich in fruit and vegetables have been proven to decrease the risk of heart attacks, strokes and a variety of cancers, and healthy, glowing skin is another by-product of eating a colourful, varied diet.

Know your portions Just because it's healthy and vegan, it doesn't mean that it can't make you gain weight. This is a common misconception when people adopt a vegan diet. Even if you stick to healthy foods, you still have to watch your portion sizes and quantities when consuming foods such as nuts, hummus, avocado, olive oil and dark chocolate (in other words, all the things marked with an asterisk in The Food Effect tables). They may be healthy but that does not mean that you can eat them freely. There's definitely a benefit in consuming a little olive oil but pouring it liberally over your pasta, and dipping your bread in it, will lead to excessive calories and weight gain. The same goes for nuts – learn what a normal serving size looks like (it's very easy to eat a whole big bag) and limit yourself to that.

The Food Effect Diet Vegan rules in brief

These rules go hand in hand with the above principles for healthy eating and weight loss. If you follow both sets of guidelines, you'll be guaranteed weight-loss success, and will look and feel better than ever. The Food Effect Diet Vegan diet is all about being the best version of you – so there are no excuses for not following these rules.

1. **Prepare, prepare, prepare** This is the golden rule of healthy eating habits. The more organised you are, the easier, and more likely, healthy eating and living will be. Make your own lunch where possible, pre-chop vegetables to have on hand for meals and snacks, and keep your fridge and cupboards stocked with the right healthy foods.

2. **Avoid highly processed and packaged foods as much as possible** Read the labels on food products – don't buy what you can't pronounce or have never heard of. As mentioned, something labelled vegan does *not* mean it's healthy.

3. **Don't go hungry** Always carry healthy snacks with you if you know you're going to be out and about for a while or working long hours. For convenience, all snacks are listed daily in your plan, and there is also a long list of options in Chapter 12, so there's really no excuse. But . . .

4. **Don't graze** Eating regularly does not mean that you should be constantly picking throughout the day. A few nuts here and there do add up. Stick to your three meals and two snacks per day – and nothing outside that. Have them whenever you feel it suits you best to do so.

5. **Ditch the white stuff** Cutting out the white stuff (think white sugar, white bread, flour, pasta and sugary, low-fibre cereals – not almond milk and cauliflower) is one of the easiest ways to lose weight and improve your health. Most processed, refined carbohydrate foods are just empty calories with little fibre and goodness.

6. **Don't cut out all starchy foods** As explained in Chapter 3, this would be a recipe for long-term diet disaster.

7. **Eat good fats** As I explained in Chapter 6, you need some good fat in order to burn fat. This means eating good, healthy unsaturated fats found in nuts, peanut butter, avocados, olive oil and various other healthy oils, as mentioned in the principles above. These are all included (in specified amounts) in the plan as they are proven to lower the risk of heart disease and aid the body in the absorption of vitamins and minerals, as well as helping with satiety, cravings and weight loss.

8. **Avoid trans fats** Often listed under the names 'hydrogenated oil' or 'hydrogenated vegetable fat', and found in many processed vegan-friendly foods, these are toxic

and have no health benefits whatsoever. Manufacturers don't have to list them if they are below 0.5g but this can mount up.

9.   **Eat vegetables and fruit** You can eat as much salad, and fresh, steamed, stir-fried and baked vegetables, as you like (within the specified meals), as long as they don't have added dressing or oil (apart from the amount specified in the plan). You can add as much lemon juice, balsamic vinegar or apple cider vinegar as you like. Fruit is also included in healthy, specified portions in the plan.

10. **Eat slowly and chew thoroughly** Take time to enjoy and savour all your food (meals and snacks). Chewing your food properly will aid efficient digestion, stop you from overeating and reduce any uncomfortable bloating you may experience from eating too quickly.

11. **Drink plenty of water** Make sure you drink 1–2 glasses of water before every meal or snack you have. If you have difficulty drinking enough plain water (around 2 litres a day), herbal teas, green tea (hot or iced) or lemon in hot water are all just as good.

12. **No sugary soft drinks or fruit juice** As explained in Chapter 3.

13. **Weigh yourself** Do this first thing in the morning, after you've gone to the toilet to empty your bladder, without any clothes on. In the Attack Phase I advise you to weigh yourself every day, for the first four weeks. The theory behind this, and why it is beneficial for weight loss, is explained in Chapter 11. After the first four weeks, once you're at the Lifestyle Phase, you should weigh yourself in the same way, once a week.

14. **Start your morning with a mug of warm water and apple cider vinegar** It's even better than warm water and lemon – often promoted as the healthiest way to start the day – so my advice is to kick off the morning with a mug of warm water and apple cider vinegar. Put a tablespoon of apple cider vinegar – a wonder food with lots of healing properties – into a mug of warm water. Drinking this will hydrate you and cleanse your digestive system. It's more effective than a probiotic, and it's the perfect way to set up your body for its daily food intake ahead, as well as helping to prevent bloating. Even though it's a vinegar it actually neutralises acid and puts your body in a good pH balance so that your internal systems work well. It can also kill bad bacteria in the stomach and intestine, and promotes good gut bacteria. I must admit that I personally struggle with the taste 'straight up' so I add a teaspoon or two of stevia or agave syrup to make it more palatable. There's absolutely no health downside to doing this, so do try it.

15. **Have a big hot drink with your breakfast (and mid-morning)** This provides a warm, comforting start to the day that, combined with a good breakfast, leaves you feeling satisfied for the day ahead. It can be tea, coffee, herbal or green tea. You can add almond or any plant-based milk with no added sugar. Sweeteners such as stevia and xylitol are allowed with no restriction (see Chapter 3).

16. **A word on caffeine** Although excess caffeine is obviously not good, caffeine from good-quality coffee (without added sugar or syrups) is packed full of antioxidants and has been shown to have tremendous health benefits. When consumed before a workout, it has also been shown to boost performance and stamina while exercising. Keep to a maximum of two coffees a day, preferably early in the day – not late afternoon or evening, so as not to disrupt your sleep.

17. **Limit (but don't shun) alcohol** There are many health benefits to alcohol as long as it's consumed in moderation, and you stick to the right choices. Drink no more than three glasses a week during the Attack Phase, and a maximum of one per night (up to seven drinks a week) once on the Lifestyle Phase. Keep to the drinks listed under 'Drink this' in the table on page 36, although it's fine to drink those in the 'Be careful' category occasionally. Sticking to this limit will help you lose weight, clear your head and improve your energy levels, without making you cut out alcohol completely. For more on alcohol, see Chapter 9.

18. **Don't give up or get despondent** We're all human and have our ups and downs. Although you are aiming to be disciplined in your food choices, The Food Effect Diet Vegan healthy-eating lifestyle is not intended to starve or deprive you. If you do slip up, it's certainly not the end of the world. Don't feel as though you've failed and then set yourself back further by going on a total binge fest – just accept it and move on.

Enjoy your Food Effect journey and remember that as long as you continue to be consistent in the process, you will reap the benefits and get fantastic results.

Tips to ensure that the changes to your healthy lifestyle last

Change your mindset Don't think of The Food Effect Diet Vegan healthy eating and weight-loss plan as a 'diet' – something that you go on and eventually come off. Reframe this as a new way of life. That way, when, or if, you do slip up, you'll be less likely to give up and get despondent because you'll realise that one or two meals (or even days), of not-too-perfect eating won't undo your overall commitment to a healthy lifestyle; you'll just get straight back to your normal healthy routine afterwards. Also, although many people start out a healthy-eating plan with a specific goal weight in mind, the real goal is to be healthy – weight loss is just a fantastic side effect – so when you do reach your weight-loss goal, you won't shift back to your old habits because it's all about feeling great.

Be realistic If you love a sweet treat or chocolate, for example, don't try to stick to a long-term healthy-eating plan thinking that you'll never have these things again. Instead, be realistic and allow for special occasions, indulgences or controlled amounts of your 'vice' food – perhaps switching to a healthier version of it (such as 70 per cent dark chocolate instead of poor-quality, sugar-laden vegan chocolate).

Set manageable goals By doing the opposite (that is, being unrealistic), you just set yourself up for failure and worse – feeling like a failure – and you are thus more likely to give up altogether. If the thought of eating a bowl of healthy greens makes you nauseous, make changes in small increments; for example, by adding one serving of fresh vegetables a day, until you're ready to push for more. Also, if you prefer to take a 'flexitarian' approach to eating, and aim to be vegan most of the time, but not always, that is totally fine and healthy, too. Don't take on anything you feel is unmanageable or too extreme.

Team up Research has shown that dieters are more successful when they have support. That might involve partnering with a friend to do The Food Effect Diet Vegan, or asking family members to encourage you and provide support. If you feel that your eating habits are tied to emotional issues (not an uncommon problem), such as loneliness, depression, and so on, consider seeking help for those issues too.

Prepare, prepare, prepare As we have seen, this is the golden rule of successful healthy eating habits. The more you think ahead and take a few moments to plan and prepare your food, the more likely and easier it will be for you to enjoy healthy and tasty food, and the less likely you will be to make unhealthy choices when going about your day, rushed in the moment. Think ahead about the food and meals you intend to eat, and make sure you have the right things on hand (you now have plenty of perfect examples and suggestions). If you're constantly on the go, that will be no excuse for unhealthy eating – just make sure you have grab-and-go options always to hand. The Food Effect Diet Vegan plan and meal options provide plenty of easy suggestions.

Perfect your shopping list If you buy good food, you'll eat good food. Similarly, if you don't buy junk food and keep it stocked at home, you'll be less likely to eat junk food altogether. Everyone in your home will benefit from this one, too. See 'Kitchen staples' (page 276) for the basics on what to have stocked.

Treat yourself with non-food rewards. Choose small rewards for reaching your goals along the way (and bigger ones for bigger goals). Try to choose a treat for yourself that will further enhance your feel-good lifestyle (such as a massage or an indulgent pampering product), or perhaps even something that will fuel it further (like some stylish workout clothing).

Make it enjoyable Make your healthful Food Effect Diet Vegan lifestyle fun and enjoyable. Try new healthy recipes, share them with friends or cook for others. Get ideas online via social media – there are loads of great nutrition blogs out there. To start with, make sure you follow @thefoodeffectdr on Instagram, and The Food Effect on Facebook, for your daily dose of inspiration. And check out www.thefoodeffect.co.uk for ongoing cooking inspiration and all the latest in nutrition.

REFERENCES

Chapter 2

Steinberg, D.M., Bennett, G.G., Askew, S., Tate, D.F., 'Weighing every day matters: Daily weighing improves weight loss and adoption of weight control behaviors', *Journal of the Academy of Nutrition and Dietetics*, 114(4) (2015), pp. 511–18

Chapter 3

Hyun-seok, Kim, 'Prevalence of celiac appears steady but followers of gluten-free diet increase', *JAMA Internal Medicine*, 6 September 2016

Jéquier, E., 'Carbohydrates as a source of energy', *American Journal of Clinical Nutrition*, (1994) (3 Suppl): pp. 682S–685S, doi: 10.1093/ajcn/59.3.682S

De Angelis, M., Rizzello, C.G., Alfonsi, G., Arnault, P., et al., 'Use of sourdough lactobacilli and oat fibre to decrease the glycaemic index of white wheat bread', *British Journal of Nutrition*, 98(6) (2007), pp. 1196–205

Poutanen, K., Flander, L., Katina, K., 'Sourdough and cereal fermentation in a nutritional perspective', *Food Microbiology*, 26(7) (2009), pp. 693–9 doi: 10.1016/j.fm.2009.07.011

Gobbetti, M., Rizzello, C.G., Di Cagno, R., De Angelis, M., 'How the sourdough may affect the functional features of leavened baked goods', *Food Microbiology*, 37 (2014), pp. 30–40. doi: 10.1016/j. fm.2013.04.012

Liljeberg, H.G., Lönner, C.H., Björck, I.M., 'Sourdough fermentation or addition of organic acids or corresponding salts to bread improves nutritional properties of starch in healthy humans', *Journal of Nutrition*, 125(6) (1995), pp. 1503–11

Maioli, M., Pes, G.M., Sanna, M., Cherchi, S., et al., 'Sourdough-leavened bread improves postprandial glucose and insulin plasma levels in subjects with impaired glucose tolerance', *Acta Diabetalogica*, 45(2) (2008), pp. 91–6, doi: 10.1007/s00592–008–0029–8

Liljeberg, H.G., Björck, I.M., 'Delayed gastric emptying rate as a potential mechanism for lowered glycemia after eating sourdough bread: Studies in humans and rats using test products with added organic acids or an organic salt', *American Journal of Clinical Nutrition*, 64(6) (1996), pp. 86–93

Kim, Hyun-seok, Patel, Kalpesh G., Orosz, Evan et al.,'Time trends in the prevalence of celiac disease and gluten-free diet in the US population: Results from the National Health and Nutrition Examination Surveys 2009–2014', *JAMA Intern Med.*, 176(11) (2016), pp. 1716–1717

Jones, A. L., 'The gluten-free diet: Fad or necessity?' *Diabetes Spectrum*, 30(2) (2017), pp. 118–23

Chapter 4

Vanga, S.K., Raghavan, V., 'How well do plant based alternatives fare nutritionally compared to cow's milk?', *Journal of Food Science and Technology*, 55(10) (2018), https://doi.org/10.1007/s13197–017–2915-y

Rial, Sabri Ahmed, et al., 'Gut microbiota and metabolic health: The potential beneficial effects of a medium chain triglyceride diet in obese individuals', *Nutrients*, 8(5) (2016) p.281, doi:10.3390/nu8050281

St-Onge, M.-P., et al., 'Impact of medium and long chain triglycerides consumption on appetite and food intake in overweight men', *European Journal of Clinical Nutrition*, 68(10) (2014), pp. 1134–40, doi:10.1038/ejcn.2014.145

Wang, Ying, et al., 'Medium chain triglycerides enhances exercise endurance through the increased mitochondrial biogenesis and metabolism', *PloS One*, vol. 13,2 (2018) 2 e0191182. doi:10.1371/journal.pone.0191182

Badger, T.M., Ronis, M.J., et al., 'Soy protein isolate and protection against cancer', *Journal of the American College of Nutrition*, 24 (2005), pp. 146S–149S

Shu, X.O., Zheng, Y., Cai, H., et al., 'Soy food intake and breast cancer survival', *JAMA*, 302(22) (2009), pp. 2437–2443, doi:10.1001/jama.2009.1783

Guha, N., Kwan, M.L., Quesenberry, C.P. Jr, et al., 'Soy isoflavones and risk of cancer recurrence in a cohort of breast cancer survivors: The Life After Cancer Epidemiology study', *Breast Cancer Research and Treatment*, 118 (2009), pp. 395–405

www.youtube.com Dr Eric Berg DC, 'Do Phytoestrogens Really Increase Your Estrogen Levels?'

Hamilton-Reeves, J.M., Vazquez, G., Duval, S.J., et al., 'Clinical studies show no effects of soy protein or isoflavones on reproductive hormones in men: Results of a meta-analysis', *Fertility and Sterility*, 94 (2010), pp. 997–1007

Yan, L., Spitznagel, E.L., 'Soy consumption and prostate cancer risk in men: A revisit of a meta-analysis', *American Journal of Clinical Nutrition*, 89 (2009), pp. 1155–63

University of Illinois at Urbana-Champaign, 'How does soy promote weight loss?' *Science Daily*, 6 May 2007, www.sciencedaily.com/releases/2007/05/070501115010.htm.

Society for the Study of Ingestive Behavior, 'Meals as medicine: Anti-obesity effects of soy in rat model of menopause', *Science Daily*, 26 July 2010, www.sciencedaily.com/releases/2010/07/100713011041.htm

NIH Website, National Center for Complementary and Integrative Health, 'Soy', https://nccih.nih.gov/health/soy/ataglance.htm

Murty, C.M., Pittaway, J.K., Ball, M.J., 'Chickpea supplementation in an Australian diet affects food choice, satiety and bowel health', *Appetite*, 54 (2010), pp. 282–88, doi: 10.1016/j.appet.2009.11.012

O'Neil, C.E., Nicklas, T.A., Fulgoni, V.L., 'Chickpeas and hummus are associated with better nutrient intake, diet quality, and levels of some cardiovascular risk factors: National Health and Nutrition Examination Survey 2003–2010', *Journal of Nutrition and Food Sciences*, 4(1) (2014), doi: 10.4172/2155–9600.1000254

Papanikolaou, Y., Fulgoni, V.L., III, 'Bean consumption is associated with greater nutrient intake, reduced systolic blood pressure, lower body weight, and a smaller waist circumference in adults: Results from the National Health and Nutrition Examination Survey 1999–2002', *Journal of the American College of Nutrition*, 27 (2008) pp. 569–76. doi: 10.1080/07315724.2008.10719740

Mitchell, D.C., Lawrence, F.R., Hartman, T.J., Curran, J.M., 'Consumption of dry beans, peas, and lentils could improve diet quality in the US population', *Journal of the Academy of Nutrition and Dietetics*, 109 (2009), pp. 909–13, doi: 10.1016/j.jada.2009.02.029

Pittaway, J.K., Robertson, I.K., Ball, M.J., 'Chickpeas may influence fatty acid and fiber intake in an ad libitum diet, leading to small improvements in serum lipid profile and glycemic control', *Journal of the American Dietetic Association*, 108 (2008), pp. 1009–13. doi: 10.1016/j.jada.2008.03.009

https://www.healthifyme.com/blog/5-reasons-raw-jackfruit-superfood/

Memisoglu, A., Hu, F.B., Hankinson, S.E., et al., 'Interaction between a peroxisome proliferator-activated receptor gamma gene polymorphism and dietary fat intake in relation to body mass', *Human Molecular Genetics*, 12(22) (2003), pp. 2923–9

Esselstyn, C.B. Jr, Gendy, G., Doyle, J., et al., 'A way to reverse CAD?', *Journal of Family Practice*, 63(7) (2014), pp. 356–364b

Vuksan, V., Jenkinsa, A.L., Brissette, C., et al., 'Salba-chia (Salvia hispanica L.) in the treatment of overweight and obese patients with type 2 diabetes: A double-blind randomized controlled trial', *Nutrition, Metabolism and Cardiovascular Diseases*, December 2016

Chapter 5

Mingyang Song, 'Eating more plant protein associated with lower risk of death', *JAMA Internal Medicine*, 1 August 2016

Bujnowski, D., Xun, P., Daviglus, M.L., et al., 'Longitudinal association between animal and vegetable protein intake and obesity among men in the United States: The Chicago Western Electric Study', *Journal of the American Dietetic Association*, 111(8) (2011), pp. 1150–55

Wang, X., Lin, X., Ouyang, Y.Y., et al., 'Red and processed meat consumption and mortality: Dose-response meta-analysis of prospective cohort studies', *Public Health Nutrition*, 19(5) (2016), pp. 893–905

Pan, A., Sun, Q., Bernstein, A.M., et al., 'Red meat consumption and mortality: Results from 2 prospective cohort studies', *Archives of Internal Medicine*, 172(7) (2012), pp. 555–63

Lagiou, P., Sandin, S., Weiderpass, E., et al., 'Low carbohydrate-high protein diet and mortality in a cohort of Swedish women', *Journal of Internal Medicine*, 261(4) (2007), pp. 366–74

Fung, T.T., van Dam, R.M., Hankinson, S.E, et al., 'Low-carbohydrate diets and all-cause and cause-specific mortality: Two cohort studies', *Annals of Internal Medicine*, 153(5) (2010), pp. 289–98

Pan, A., Sun, Q., Bernstein, A.M., et al., 'Changes in red meat consumption and subsequent risk of type-2 diabetes mellitus: Three cohorts of US men and women', *JAMA Internal Medicine*, 173(14) (2013), pp. 1328–35

Morris, M.C., Evans, D.A., Bienias, J.L., et al., 'Dietary fats and the risk of incident Alzheimer disease', *Archives of Neurology*, 60(2) (2003), pp. 194–200

Richman, E.L, Kenfield, S.A., Stampfer, M.J., et al., 'Choline intake and risk of lethal prostate cancer: Incidence and survival', *American Journal of Clinical Nutrition*, 96(4) (2012), pp. 855–63

Ornish, D., Magbanua, M.J., Weidner, G., et al., 'Changes in prostate gene expression in men undergoing an intensive nutrition and lifestyle intervention', *Proceedings of the National Academy of Sciences USA*, 105(24) (2008), pp. 8369–74

Parazzini, F., Viganò, P., Candiani, M., Fedele, L., 'Diet and endometriosis risk: A literature review', *American Journal of Obstetrics and Gynecology*, 26(4) (2013), pp. 323–36

Lewis, S.J., Heaton, K.W., Oakey, R.E., McGarrigle, H.H., 'Lower serum oestrogen concentrations associated with faster intestinal transit', *British Journal of Cancer*, 76(3) (1997), pp. 395–400

Alexander, D.D., Morimoto, L.M., Mink, P.J., et al., 'A review and meta-analysis of red and processed meat consumption and breast cancer', *Nutrition Research Reviews*, 23(2) (2010), pp. 349–65

Ping-Ping Bao, Xiao-Ou Shu, Ying Zheng, et al., 'Fruit, vegetable, and animal food intake and breast cancer risk by hormone receptor status', *Nutrition and Cancer*, 64(6) (2012), pp. 806–19

National Cancer Institute, 'Chemicals in meat cooked at high temperatures and cancer risk', https://www.cancer.gov/about-cancer/causes-prevention/risk/diet/cooked-meats-fact-sheet

Frattaroli, J., Weidner, G., Merritt-Worden, T.A., et al., 'Angina pectoris and atherosclerotic risk factors in the multisite cardiac lifestyle intervention programme', *American Journal of Cardiology*, 101(7) (2008), pp. 911–18

Chapter 6

de Gaetano, G., 'Mediterranean diet associated with lower risk of early death in cardiovascular disease patients', *European Society of Cardiology*, 29 August 2016

Morris, M.C., Evans, D.A., Bienias, J.L., et al., 'Dietary fats and the risk of incident Alzheimer's disease', *Archives of Neurology*, 60(2) (2003), pp. 194–200

Endocrine Society, 'To reduce body fat, eating less fat may be more effective than eating less carbohydrate', *Science Daily*, 5 March 2015, www.sciencedaily.com/releases/2015/03/150305151834.htm

Memisoglu, A., Hu, F.B., Hankinson, S.E., et al., 'Interaction between a peroxisome proliferator-activated receptor gamma gene polymorphism and dietary fat intake in relation to body mass', *Human Molecular Genetics*,12(22) (2003), pp. 2923–9

Wien, M., Haddad, E., Oda, K,. Sabaté, J., 'A randomized 3×3 crossover study to evaluate the effect of Hass avocado intake on post-ingestive satiety, glucose and insulin levels, and subsequent energy intake in overweight adults', *Nutrition Journal*, 12 (2013), no. 155

Chapter 7

Wallace, T.C., Murray, R., Zelman, K.M., 'The nutritional value and health benefits of chickpeas and hummus', *Nutrients*, 8(12) (2016), p. 766, doi:10.3390/nu8120766

Murty, C.M., Pittaway, J.K., Ball, M.J., 'Chickpea supplementation in an Australian diet affects food choice, satiety and bowel health', *Appetite*, 54 (2010) pp. 282–8, doi: 10.1016/j.appet.2009.11.012

Jukanti, A., Gaur, P., Gowda, C., Chibbar, R., 'Nutritional quality and health benefits of chickpea (Cicer arietinum L.): A review', *British Journal of Nutrition*, 108(S1) (2012), S11–S26, doi:10.1017/S0007114512000797

Papanikolaou, Y., Fulgoni, V.L., III, 'Bean consumption is associated with greater nutrient intake, reduced systolic blood pressure, lower body weight, and a smaller waist circumference in adults: Results from the National Health and Nutrition Examination Survey 1999–2002', *Journal of the American College of Nutrition*, 27 (2008), pp. 569–576, doi: 10.1080/07315724.2008.10719740

O'Neil, C.E., Nicklas, T.A., Fulgoni, V.L., 'Chickpeas and hummus are associated with better nutrient intake, diet quality, and levels of some cardiovascular risk factors: National Health and Nutrition Examination Survey 2003–2010', *Journal of Nutrition and Food Sciences*, 4 (20140 p. 1, doi: 10.4172/2155–9600.1000254,

Pittaway, J.K., Robertson, I.K., Ball, M.J., 'Chickpeas may influence fatty acid and fiber intake in an ad libitum diet, leading to small improvements in serum lipid profile and glycemic control', *Journal of the American Dietetic Association*, 108 (2008) pp. 1009–13, doi: 10.1016/j.jada.2008.03.009

Soutschek, A., Ruff, C.C., Strombach, T., et al., 'Brain stimulation reveals crucial role of overcoming self-centeredness in self-control', *Science Advances*, 2(10) (2016), e1600992, doi: 10.1126/sciadv.1600992

Chapter 9

Rasouli, B., Ahlbom, A., Andersson, T., et al., 'Alcohol consumption is associated with reduced risk of Type 2 diabetes and autoimmune diabetes in adults: Results from the Nord-Trøndelag health study'. *Diabetic Medicine*, 30(1) (2013), pp. 56–64

Berkey, C.S., et al., 'Weight gain in older adolescent females: The Internet, sleep, coffee, and alcohol', *Journal of Pediatrics*, 153(5) (2008), p. 639

Gruchow, H.W., et al., 'Alcohol consumption, nutrient intake and relative body weight among US adults', *American Journal of Clinical Nutrition*, 42 (1985), pp. 289–95

Arif, A.A., Rohrer, J.E., 'Patterns of alcohol drinking and its association with obesity: Data from the third national health and nutrition examination survey 1988–1994', *BMC Public Health*, 5(5) (2005), p. 126

Wang, L. et al., 'Alcohol consumption, weight gain, and risk of becoming overweight in middle-aged and older women', *Archives of Internal Medicine*, 170(5) (2010), pp. 453–61

Lahti-Koski, M., et al., 'Associations of body mass index and obesity with physical activity, food choices, alcohol intake, and smoking in the 1982–1997 FINRISK studies', *American Journal of Clinical Nutrition*, 75(5) (2002), pp. 809–17

Chapter 10

Malhotra, A., Noakes, T., Phinney, S., 'It is time to bust the myth of physical inactivity and obesity: You cannot outrun a bad diet', *British Journal of Sports Medicine*, 49 (2015), pp. 967–8

Pereira, A., Huddleston, D., Brickman, A., et al., 'An in vivo correlate of exercise-induced neurogenesis in the adult dentate gyrus', *Proceedings of the National Academy of Sciences USA*, 104(13) (2007), pp. 5638–43

Ornish, D., Lin, J., Chan, J. M., et al., 'Effect of comprehensive lifestyle changes on telomerase activity and telomere length in men with biopsy-proven low-risk prostate cancer: 5-year follow-up of a descriptive pilot study', *Lancet Oncology*, 14(11) (2013), pp. 1112–20

Frattaroli, J., Weidner, G., Merritt-Worden, T. A., et al., 'Angina pectoris and atherosclerotic risk factors in the multisite cardiac lifestyle intervention program', *American Journal of Cardiology*, 101(7) (2008), pp. 911–18

Craig, B.W., Brown, R., Everhart, J., 'Effects of progressive resistance training on growth hormone and testosterone levels in young and elderly subjects', *Mechanisms of Ageing and Development*, 49(2) (1989), pp. 159–69

Hamilton, L.D., Fogle, E.A., Meston, C.M., 'The roles of testosterone and alpha-amylase in exercise-induced sexual arousal in women', *Journal of Sexual Medicine*, 5 (2008), pp. 845–53

Samji, V., Haykal, T., Zayed, Y., et al., 'Role of vitamin D supplementation for primary prevention of cancer: Meta-analysis of randomized controlled trials', *Journal of Clinical Oncology*, 37 (15_suppl) (2019) 1534, doi:10.1200/JCO.2019.37.15_suppl.1534

'Everyone should take vitamin D pills, doctors warn', *The Times*, 21 July 2016

Wing, R.R., Phelan, S. 'Long-term weight loss maintenance', *American Journal of Clinical Nutrition*, 82(1) (2005), pp. 222S–225S.

Chapter 11

Steinberg, D.M., Bennett, G.G., Askew, S., Tate, D.F., 'Weighing every day matters: Daily weighing improves weight loss and adoption of weight control behaviors', *Journal of the Academy of Nutrition and Dietetics*, 114(4) (2015), pp. 511–18

INDEX

ACKNOWLEDGEMENTS

My deepest thanks to my most incredible literary agent, Heather Holden-Brown of hhb Agency, who has supported me from book one to book two. Heather, you had faith in me from day one, when the first *The Food Effect Diet* book was just an idea in my head. Your constant guidance, support and unwavering encouragement enabled me to make my dreams a reality, for not just one book but two.

Thank you to everyone at Little, Brown for making this book everything that it is. A special thank-you to Zoe Bohm and Jillian Stewart, who gave me invaluable editorial guidance and supported me every step along the way. You are both beyond thorough and talented at everything you do, and it's been such a privilege to work with you now on two books. Thank you to Hannah Wood for coordinating and putting together the cover design, and to Beth Wright for all your hard work in coordinating the PR for the book.

Thank you to Liron Weissman and Aviva Soloman for your incredible skills and talent in creating the cover photograph for both my books.

Thank you to the amazing and inspiring Rachida Brocklehurst for writing the wonderful Foreword for this book.

Thank you to my amazing Mom and Dad – there are no

words to express my love for you both or my gratitude for everything you have done, and continue to do, for me. You are my role models in every aspect of life, and you have supported me in everything I do since the day I was born. Thank you to my amazing brother and sister, siblings-in-law, family and friends for always being there for me. I love you all so much.

Thank you to the love of my life, my husband, Jeff. There are no words to express how much I love and adore you, and how much you brighten up my life. You encourage and support me with my work and ambitions, and are always there to inspire me to achieve my dreams. Thank you for being my rock in everything I do always.

Finally, thank you so much to all my clients, past and present – I'd never have gained all the knowledge and insight into successful weight loss and how people deal with eating, dieting and life, without all of you. You've all inspired me so much.

Thank you so much.

Michelle xx